FAIL-PROOF GUIDE TO VEGAN BODYBUILDING AND FITNESS

Discover Everything You Must Know About Plant-Based Bodybuilding in Just 7 Days... Even if You're a Brand New Vegan Athlete

BRAD SPEER

© **Copyright 2020 by Priscilla Posey - All rights reserved.**

The content contained within this book may not be reproduced, duplicated or transmitted without direct written permission from the author or the publisher.

Under no circumstances will any blame or legal responsibility be held against the publisher, or author, for any damages, reparation, or monetary loss due to the information contained within this book. Either directly or indirectly.

Legal Notice:

This book is copyright protected. This book is only for personal use. You cannot amend, distribute, sell, use, quote or paraphrase any part, or the content within this book, without the consent of the author or publisher.

Disclaimer Notice:

Please note the information contained within this document is for educational and entertainment purposes only. All effort has been executed to present accurate, up to date, and reliable, complete information. No warranties of any kind are declared or implied. Readers acknowledge that the author is not engaging in the rendering of legal, financial, medical or professional advice. The content within this book has been derived from various sources. Please consult a licensed professional before attempting any techniques outlined in this book.

By reading this document, the reader agrees that under no circumstances is the author responsible for any losses, direct or indirect, which are incurred as a result of the use of the information contained within this document, including, but not limited to, — errors, omissions, or inaccuracies.

👀 Look! Special Offer Currently Available! 👀

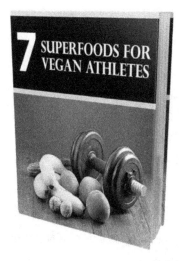

⚠ Warning: Downloads of this book have been limited to 15 FREE Downloads. Then, the price instantly shoots up to $27 ⚠

Hurry! Get Your Copy Now by Clicking the Link Below:

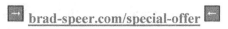

brad-speer.com/special-offer

Here's just a fraction of what you'll discover:

- 7 secret superfoods that you had NO IDEA existed!
- A secret superfood to increase the release of testosterone!
- How these foods can enhance your overall health and build muscle too!

...and so much more!!

Table of Contents

Introduction vii

Chapter 1: Bodybuilding Basics You NEED to Know 1

    So You Decided to Be a Vegan? 3

    Being a Complete Bodybuilder, Mentally and Physically 14

    Bodybuilding Basics 17

    Summary 38

Chapter 2: Fail-Proof Strategies to ELIMINATE the Most Common Excuses People Have and Defeat Limiting Beliefs So that YOU Can Get Results Fast! 41

    How to Stay Motivated With the Vegan Lifestyle 42

    How to Stay Motivated with Bodybuilding 46

    Apps to Help You Stay Motivated 50

    Finding a Workout Partner 54

    Exercise Equals Happiness 58

    Why Bodybuilders Must Master Meditation 60

Vanquishing Common Excuses For Not Going To The Gym . 63

Dispel Toxic Beliefs on Vegan Bodybuilding 66

Summary 69

Chapter 3: Nutrition Secrets Revealed For Vegan Bodybuilders... Even If You're on a Tight Budget or Pressed for Time 73

What and When to Eat as a Vegan Bodybuilder 78

All About Calories 86

Everything You Need to Know About Macros and Micros ... 90

How to Plan Your Meals While on a Budget 97

Summary 102

Chapter 4: You're At the Gym... Now What Do You Do? 105

How to Choose the Best Gym 106

Gym Etiquette 113

Compound vs Isolation Exercises 116

Sample Training Program 123

Training on the Go 129

Rest Days 131

Summary 134

Chapter 5: Bodybuilding Contest Basics 135
- Which Contests Should You Join? 136
- The Show is Finished... Now What? 139
- Summary 141

Chapter 6: Lifestyle and FAQs About Vegan Bodybuilding 143
- Summary 161

Conclusion 163

References 167

INTRODUCTION

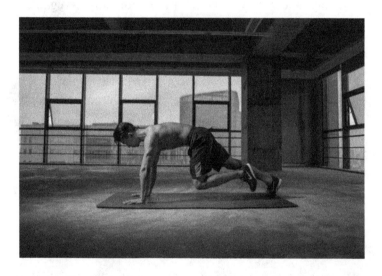

"I thought I was healthy and strong before, but after adopting a plant-based diet I started to feel energetic and I was having quicker recovery after training"
—***Frank Medrano***

So, you decided to go vegan and get into bodybuilding, but you aren't sure where to begin. You're probably questioning your decisions and wondering whether you will be able to obtain enough protein from a plant-based diet. Or maybe you're struggling with nutrition and having a hard time at the gym. Bodybuilding and veganism can go hand in hand perfectly, however, you need the right up-to-date knowledge to get started.

In this book, I will enlighten you about going vegan the right way, and help you switch from being a non-vegan to being a vegan bodybuilder. In addition, if you're completely new to bodybuilding, no problem! This book is also a complete guide to bodybuilding, and it will provide you with meal plans, as well as workout plans no matter your budget. All it takes is seven days to get started and becoming a vegan bodybuilder. By the end of this book you will know which foods you need to consume in order to gain all the rich nutrients a bodybuilder needs, and you will learn all about the challenges you will face and overcome.

Personally, I have reached my peak physique with the help of a vegan lifestyle and I have trained over 150 men and women on how to achieve the same results. Some of my clients were either beginner bodybuilders, vegans, or

Introduction

both. Others were professional bodybuilders looking to change their lifestyle and go vegan. Working with vegans as well as bodybuilders in order to help them achieve their goals is what I love doing! I grew up in a vegetarian household, so I learned about the importance of our natural environment and health from a young age. This is the main reason why I became a personal trainer. I wanted to help people better themselves.

Once you have applied the knowledge from this guide, you will achieve a strong, muscular form, as well as a healthy vegan lifestyle. In essence, you will increase your muscle mass while at the same time losing enough fat in order to reveal the muscles. Both men and women from diverse backgrounds and various ages have appreciated my training as it helped them reach their goals. Some of them went on to compete professionally in bodybuilding competitions. The training I used with them is what I want to unveil in this book. Without my help and expertise, you might learn outdated concepts, or even made up ideas that aren't reinforced by scientific evidence. You might end up eating the wrong things, doing the wrong exercises and setting yourself back due to improper knowledge. What's worse is that you might seriously injure yourself. That is why you need to learn things correctly from a solid source.

This vegan guide to bodybuilding has already yielded great results for men and women of different ages and with various degrees of experience. Each chapter will contain useful information that can be immediately applied. Learn the secrets behind increasing your muscle mass, while also eliminating animal products from your diet. By investing in this book and using the knowledge inside it, you will improve yourself without a doubt and you will reach any goals you set to achieve.

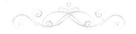

CHAPTER 1

Bodybuilding Basics You NEED to Know

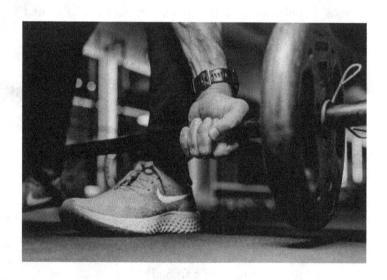

Combining a vegan diet with bodybuilding is becoming one of the most popular ways to get fit while also maintaining a healthy lifestyle. However, there are still many bodybuilders and fitness enthusiasts that are skeptical when it comes to eliminating meat from their diet while attempting to build muscle mass. Let's start this first chapter by dispelling the false image of the vegan diet.

There's a common misconception that you can't develop your muscles and you can't gain much strength without eating meat and other animal products. It is true that most bodybuilders rely on meat, dairy products, and various supplements that contain ingredients obtained from animals. However, they don't build their muscle mass and get fit purely because of consuming animal products. The main ingredient that bodybuilders are after is protein, which is found in meat, dairy products and nearly any other dietary item that is sourced from animals. Fortunately, protein can also be found in various plants, but many people aren't aware of it, or they believe that the protein content is too low to matter. Again, this is a misconception. A plant-based diet can be planned in such a way to provide you with all the protein and other nutrients you need to obtain a fit body.

Diet is key to bodybuilding and becoming fit in general. However, it needs to be combined with the correct exercises that will suit your goals. People choose bodybuilding as a lifestyle, or exercise regimen, for different reasons. Some of them like to work hard and sculpt their bodies into temples, while others simply pursue a healthier way of life. No matter the reasons, the lifestyle of a bodybuilder is something you will never regret.

With that being said, in the following sections, we are going to explore the world of bodybuilding and discuss the basics you need to know in order to get started. You will also learn about the vegan diet and how it differs from the diet of a meat-eating bodybuilder.

So You Decided to Be a Vegan?

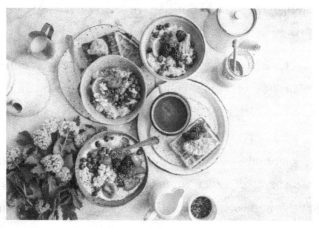

First of all, congratulations are in order because making the decision to become vegan and actually taking this step is difficult and it changes a lot of things about your lifestyle. Living a cruelty-free life isn't easy, but even if that was the only pro-veganism argument, it would still provide you with a good enough reason to make the change. Changing your life to the benefit of your health, those around you, and nature itself can be extremely empowering and motivating on its own. Going vegan and avoiding animal-related products come with many benefits. For instance, by accepting a diet centered around plants you will most likely improve your body's energy levels, as well as cholesterol levels. This lifestyle comes with many new perks and even opportunities will allow you to explore different facets of life. With that being said, here are the reasons why you should go fully vegan if you haven't already done so, or if you have only taken the first step:

1. Cruelty towards animals: Animal cruelty is a huge issue, especially with an ever-increasing human population. New farms need to be built and farmers need to constantly increase the number of animals they are breeding and raising in a limited space in order to face increasing demands. By going vegan you will contribute to solving this

problem and reduce the number of suffering animals.

2. Sustainability: Related to the aforementioned issue, increasing the world's meat consumption is also a natural disaster on its own. With the increasing global population, forests need to be cleared to make room for farmland in order to breed more animals for human consumption and to create various products. This is damaging to nature and we can already see its negative effects today as this problem significantly contributes to global warming. Eating a plant-based diet and giving up on animal byproducts is a sustainable, long-term solution that will benefit future generations and nature itself.

3. Social impact: Going vegan is partially about impacting nature and society in a positive way. By joining a group of people who think alike, your personal impact on nature will have a greater meaning because it is easier to make significant changes when part of a community.

4. Avoiding health-risks: Several of the largest modern health problems today are caused by a bad diet. Many people suffer from clogged arteries,

obesity, various heart problems, diabetes and so on. Most of these hazards can be avoided by switching to a plant-based diet.

5. More energy and focus: Plant-based diets are rich in vitamins, fatty acids, amino acids, and carbohydrates, in addition to protein and healthy fats. All of these ingredients are essential to a healthy life, not just for building muscle mass. Through a vegan diet, you will notice that you will start waking up fresher than ever before and have more energy throughout your day.

While a plant-based diet comes with many health benefits and advantages, we cannot ignore the drawbacks. Another popular misconception that keeps people away from this lifestyle is that the diet cannot provide you with everything your body demands. This misconception stems from real shortcomings of a plant-based diet which can be fixed with the right knowledge. That is why it is important to know the drawbacks in the first place so they can easily be avoided. Keep in mind that no matter the diet you plan for yourself, you need to know what you put in your body and what it does to you. Food isn't just food that keeps you alive.

With that being said, let's take a look at the disadvantages of a vegan diet and see what we can do about them:

1. Nutrient deficiency: This is a real concern and one of the reasons why many avoid a plant-based diet. Many vegans are missing out on important nutrients, but that is because they don't learn what each plant, vegetable or fruit contains. It is important to know and understand what your body needs and where you can get it. For instance, one of the biggest issues vegans have is caused by the simple fact that they consume only common products like rice, in order to fill themselves. This way they gain a lot of carbohydrates but not enough vitamins and minerals. Another issue is that, depending on your area, it may be difficult to purchase certain plant-based products that contain calcium, iron, and Omega 3, which are nutrients normally found in various meats, fish and dairy products. Fortunately, you can easily fix this problem by taking natural supplements. For instance, Omega-3 isn't found only in fish like salmon. You can also obtain it from algae, or supplements that are made from algae. Educating

yourself on nutrition is important, especially when it comes to bodybuilding and vegan diets.

2. Proteins: Since bodybuilding and fortifying your muscle mass demands a substantial amount of protein, many bodybuilders wrongly avoid the vegan lifestyle thinking that it cannot provide enough of this essential nutrient. Keep in mind that this can be true if the diet isn't planned properly. Many vegetables and plants do not offer any protein. However, there are others that will provide you with as much as meat. For instance, beans, peas, and lentils are only a couple of food items that will offer you enough protein. All you need is proper knowledge about what you need to eat in order to gain enough protein.

3. Calories: Another issue some vegans are confronted with is either the lack of enough calories or too many of them. In order to increase your muscle mass, you need enough calories. The problem with plants is that most of them offer significantly fewer calories than animal products. This means that you need to carefully plan your diet in order to meet the required number of calories that will promote your growth and

development. This problem can again be easily fixed by knowing which foods offer the right nutritional values. The other side of the coin however, is eating vegan-friendly foods that contain too many calories and not enough essential nutrients. For instance, it is easy to eat a lot of grains and rice to meet your caloric demand. However, they will mostly provide you with carbohydrates and barely any minerals, vitamins and protein. We will discuss more about this problem when we get to the section about nutrients.

4. Boring meals: If you're someone who loves food and loves to cook, the vegan diet might be scary at first because of the dietary restrictions. The typical western diet is rich in flavors and very diverse, while plant-based diets are rarely popular because of the seemingly "boring" ingredients. After all, not many kids choose broccoli over bacon. Fortunately, your vegan meals don't have to be boring. It is fairly easy to be creative with the ingredients you consume and you can combine so many of them to create new, exciting dishes. There is no limit to what you can do with hundreds of vegetables, fruits, and herbs.

Becoming a vegan is all about being knowledgeable about the human body and the nutrients offered by a plant-based diet. Without the right knowledge, it is easy to make the wrong decisions regarding your health. This is why it is important to discuss diet in regards to bodybuilding and we will focus more on this topic in later sections.

What I Wish Someone Told Me When I First Became Vegan

As mentioned earlier, many problems stem from a lack of knowledge. It's easy to overlook various aspects of the new lifestyle when starting out. So, let's take a step back and talk a bit about the finer details in order to dispel some of the most common concerns:

1. Lack of vegan options: This is a common concern that is not true. There may be some restaurants and diners that don't offer any vegan options, but they are rare. In the U.S and in the Western world, in general, there are many vegan-only restaurants that are very imaginative with their meals. In addition, you are also free to use your creativity to create new meals in your own kitchen. There are so many ingredients available to you that you should never run out of ideas.

2. The fine print: Many vegans become a bit obsessed with the label's fine print when purchasing a vegan product. This is only normal, especially when you're just starting out because there are so many nutritional values and other details you need to pay attention to. One of the issues here is regarding the allergen warnings. There are many products out there that you might think aren't truly vegan, even when they are sold as such, because their label says "may contain milk or eggs". Please keep in mind that this warning doesn't mean the product actually contains these ingredients. It is a warning about very specific allergens found in these food items because some people have life-threatening allergies.

3. Vegan food that isn't labeled as vegan: A lot of foods are ignored by vegans, whether in restaurants or at the supermarket, simply because they aren't labeled as vegan specifically. Keep in mind that lacking the vegan label doesn't mean that a product isn't vegan. There are many products that are consumed by everyone regularly, and they just happen to be vegan. This is why you should always read the list of ingredients and not

just search for the vegan label. If the ingredients themselves are plant-based, then you can eat the product without any worries.

4. Beware of influencers: When starting a new diet or a lifestyle, most people look for some "idols" or knowledgeable people to follow or even mimic. This is especially true when it comes to fitness, bodybuilding and lifestyle changes in general. Therefore, you might be tempted to follow a certain YouTube or Instagram influencer's diet purely because you love their look and you want to achieve it as well. This is usually a mistake. You have to keep in mind that you don't know all the details about an influencer's personal life. You don't even know for certain that they respect the diet they are advertising. So, take everything you hear from them with a grain of salt. They may have had other help in achieving their looks and you will never know about it.

5. Treating non-vegans with respect: One of the reasons why veganism has a tarnished image is due to the way some vegans treat those who eat meat and other animal products. Behaving with hostility towards family and friends who refuse to

give up meat and follow a vegan diet will not help them change their minds and will also not help you gain any respect. On the contrary, such hostility will only create more hostility and create a worse image of veganism in their minds. This is why you should respect their own boundaries and only seek to discuss the topic in a friendly manner if they are open to it. Don't try to be pushy, or you will meet resistance. Simply respect them and seek to occasionally teach them what you learned, but in a non-patronizing way. This way you will discover that people are in general open to trying new things if they are presented as interesting and fun. People around you will start trying various vegan dishes and add them to their own diets. This will at the very least reduce the amount of meat and animal-derived products they consume, which is already a victory for their own health as well as the health of the environment.

Take these tips as a few simple guidelines as you integrate your new habits into your personal and professional life. To quickly summarize, all you need to do is learn how to pay attention to what you eat and respect those around you who may have different views and opinions on your new lifestyle.

Now that we briefly discussed the vegan diet side of the equation, let's start talking about bodybuilding.

Being a Complete Bodybuilder, Mentally and Physically

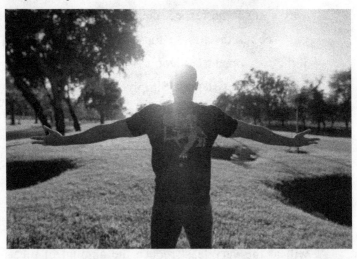

Before we dig into the basics of bodybuilding training, nutrition and so on, we need to clear up a few things about this activity.

The first thing you need to keep in mind is that bodybuilding isn't easy and you need to do it by the book (generally speaking), or as close as you can. This is not a typical sport. You don't just train for it and then compete in an event. You can't just go to the gym, do your thing, and then go home. Bodybuilding sticks to you. It is a lifestyle. You can't just drop it like a baseball bat when you're done with it at the end of the day. That is why if you do not do things properly, bodybuilding will not be enjoyable but frustrating instead.

Secondly, you need to train yourself mentally as well, not just physically. You need to become a complete bodybuilder in order to live a well-balanced, fruitful life as an individual and as a bodybuilder as well. As mentioned, you live this sport every day even when you aren't training hard at the gym. Bodybuilders aren't judged or evaluated by some regular sports criteria. Instead, we are judged by our looks. It's all about accomplishing the perfect human form. This is important to be aware of, even if you don't plan to go professional at some point, because it is easy to become obsessed with your appearance.

All people are in some ways aware of their own image and constantly worried about how they can make themselves look better. However, bodybuilders tend to become obsessed with their image. It is normal to rigidly plan every meal and time them appropriately instead of eating for pleasure. Food becomes nothing more than fuel that needs to satisfy the need for nutrients in order to build muscle mass and achieve the perfect definition. The problem is that we already talked about how the focus on the vegan diet can become overwhelming at times and many vegans become obsessed with food. If you develop that kind of mentality towards the diet, and then you add the same kind of thinking to bodybuilding, you will end up creating a recipe for disaster. You will always feel overworked, frustrated and never truly satisfied. This is why you need to prepare yourself psychologically, be aware of these things, and make sure to take baby steps when making such significant changes in your life.

The aforementioned obsession that many bodybuilders suffer from is something that psychologists call muscle dysmorphia. This is actually similar to anorexia, but the other way around. It is a condition that makes people feel small, no matter how much they grow in mass, they never feel that they have achieved the physique they were looking for. Whenever a bodybuilder is close to reaching his or her goal, that goal will move further before being reached. This is what causes a perpetual cycle of feeling inadequate. It is like chasing the pot of gold at the end of the rainbow. So take note of it right now and set your goals in stone. Do not move them forward without truly reaching them. Take baby steps and learn to appreciate yourself whenever you hit a goal no matter how small.

After all, a house is built one brick at a time, so celebrate each one of those bricks when building your temple.

Bodybuilding Basics

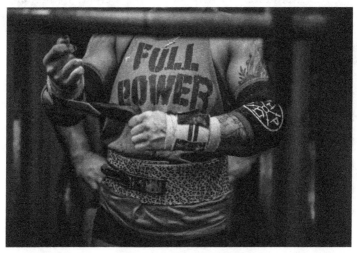

Above all else, bodybuilding requires time and dedication. You need to invest yourself in mastering the basics and be patient with yourself. Progress doesn't happen overnight. Depending on your long-term goal, it can take you months or even years to reach the desired physique. This is why in the previous section we discussed setting smaller, short-term goals for yourself. Otherwise, you will risk feeling frustrated for taking so long to achieve your end goal.

With that being said, you need to start with the basics. Bodybuilding requires a mastery of a number of different aspects.

The first thing you will need to do is create a schedule and dedicate yourself to it. Keep in mind that a workout routine isn't about repeating the same exercises every single day at a specific hour. It's all about sticking to your goals and dedicating yourself to training consistently. This takes discipline and you might need some time to adjust to this change in your life. Having a workout schedule means that rain or shine, you need to hit the gym. You don't feel like working out? You're tired from work? Or you're just feeling down? It doesn't matter, you have to reach the gym and do your exercises or you will never reach your goals. No matter what happens, you need to make the time whether it's an hour before work or an hour at midnight.

This discipline will also benefit you when it comes to your diet. A vegan diet requires willpower and planning on its own. However, this is especially important when you also add in the bodybuilding element. Nutrition is as important as lifting weights because without eating properly your body won't be able to grow no matter how much you exercise. Eating right is key and many bodybuilders end up spending more time in the kitchen making sure they eat right than at the gym.

Once you find your iron will and the right diet, you need to learn the basics of exercising. There are many modern tools out there that advertise themselves as a quick way to gaining toned muscles but they're mostly just mumbo jumbo. You need to learn the key power exercises that require nothing but your own body weight and some iron. These basic exercises will form the base of your training regimen, and they will include bench presses, deadlifts, bicep curls, dips, lateral raises, military presses, squats and so much more. There's no need to have access to fancy machines. You need some weights and together with the proper form, you will start developing your muscles and strength. Furthermore, the keyword here is 'form'. Without proper form, you will not exercise the right muscle groups or you can risk injury. So, make sure you get the basics right before you start pushing your body to its limit. We'll discuss this topic in more detail later.

Going back to your nutrition program, again, you need to learn the basics and improve your diet as you progress. The basics are fairly simple, whether you're a vegan or not. You need to eat a lot of green vegetables and enough fruit to make sure your body absorbs all the minerals and vitamins it needs. In addition, you need to consume enough calories and protein for your muscles to burn during their healing process, so that they can grow and become stronger. Keep in mind that if you aren't consuming enough calories, your body won't burn just the fat deposits in order to compensate. When there's a caloric deficit, the human body will also consume muscle tissue in order to obtain all the energy and nutrients it needs. And that is the last thing you want to happen when your goal is to grow your muscles.

As discussed earlier, protein is crucial and it is not an issue for vegans unless they fail to learn the nutritional values of what they eat. Protein isn't found in meat and dairy products alone. You can gain it from a variety of nuts and seeds, beans, tofu, soy products, as well as vegan-friendly protein supplements. Another key aspect of your basic bodybuilding diet, however, is water. Far too many beginners ignore this, but you need to drink a lot of water, especially as a bodybuilder. This is what brings all the healthy nutrients to your cells in order to energize your body more efficiently.

By now you might start seeing a pattern in bodybuilding. The key element here is efficiency. The human body is a complex machine and you need to give it what it needs to operate at peak efficiency. This means that there's also such a thing as too much. You don't want to stuff yourself with too much food, and you don't need to spend hours and hours at the gym to fulfill your goals. All you need to do is give yourself what is needed to function efficiently. Don't overdo it, because there is such a thing as too much. For instance, if you train for too long at the gym, your muscles will tear faster than they can recover. This alone can lead to injuries along the way, and they can be rather painful. All you really need is an hour, up to an hour and a half to do a full workout. Keep in mind that this also includes short resting periods between sets of exercises, which can range anywhere between half a minute to three minutes. Both the workout time as well as the breaks depend on which muscle groups you are exercising that day.

Another key component of bodybuilding is supplementation. Because diet plays such a vital role in bodybuilding, supplements are sometimes necessary as it is difficult to always get all the right nutrients you need. Keep in mind that no matter the diet you choose, it's not easy to be supplement-free. However, all you really need to stick to are the basics. Protein is the most important and popular bodybuilding supplement because it is the main building block. Most bodybuilders who eat right will also take a protein shake in the morning and one after a workout or before bedtime. Just keep in mind that supplements aren't meant to replace any of your dietary needs. They are in addition to everything else. Multivitamins are also a popular supplement taken by most bodybuilders. Your daily vegan diet may sometimes lead to various deficiencies, especially if certain food items are difficult to come by in your area. In this case, vitamin supplements are a great option, especially if you buy them in liquid form because your body can absorb them faster that way. Another frequently used supplement is an amino acid called L-Glutamine. This is an important nutrient that helps your muscles recover at a faster rate than they would normally through diet alone. Other supplements like Omega-3, Vitamin C, and many more are used, but for now, you should stick to the basics and follow a solid dietary plan.

As a bodybuilder who's just starting out, setting a number of goals is also one of the basics. Training yourself without motivation isn't fun and you might quit due to a lack of it. Therefore, you should find something that pushes you onwards. Bodybuilders need to push themselves to their physical limits and without willpower and raw determination they can rarely go the extra mile.

For most people, it's enough to just imagine how fit, strong and muscular they will be. This is enough to keep them motivated to push through the physical pain and dietary restrictions. However, no matter what your goals are, you must motivate yourself and learn what drives you. Be specific, write everything down to remind yourself months or even years later about why you even started. This is a demanding sport where mind over matter does indeed dominate.

Finally, a successful bodybuilder needs to embrace the lifestyle itself. Remember that bodybuilding isn't just a sport. You don't just train for competitions or for the sake of training itself. It is a way of life and it will impact most facets of your personal and professional life. Bodybuilding will teach you discipline, and it will keep you motivated in life. However, to achieve all of this, you need to make a series of decisions. You need to learn how to go to bed at the right time to get enough sleep so that your body can recover before the next training session. Meal preparation is another area that requires discipline and determination because you must provide your body with all the nutrients it needs to grow and stay healthy at peak performance. You need to respect your workout schedule and always make enough time to go to the gym no matter how busy you think you are.

Preparing yourself and learning all the basics from the start will give you a significant advantage over those who simply jump in. Don't be like someone who makes a New Year's resolution, heads to the gym, realizes it's difficult and even painful, and then quits. All of that happens due to a lack of preparation, both mentally and physically. So make sure to focus on the basics so that you are efficient when it comes to exercising as well as nutrition. Once you master the basics, no goal is far from reach.

The Basic Program

As mentioned earlier, before getting started you need to identify your goals. Naturally, achieving them will take a long time. Even the more moderate goals can take a year to accomplish. Sculpting the human body isn't easy, so make sure you are comfortable with this idea. You cannot allow yourself to have false expectations. However, as long as you are consistent in your training and nutrition, you will eventually accomplish what you set out to do. With that being said, as a beginner, you should stick to the basics for at least a year, possibly two. Once you go through the basic bodybuilding training, you will have enough knowledge and experience to create new goals for yourself and be better able to adapt your diet and training in order to meet them.

First, you need to consider nutrition. For a bodybuilder, the most important element in nutrition is protein. No matter how you prepare your diet, your body will need to consume around 1.5 grams of protein for every pound of your bodyweight. When you calculate the daily protein requirement however, you need to consider the fact that the average person will not absorb more than around 30 grams of protein per meal. Therefore, you can't just take all the daily protein in one go, because anything that is more than what your body can process will simply be eliminated.

Once you have the protein intake settled, you need to look at your goals in order to consider how many calories per day you need to consume. If you're a typical bodybuilder starting out with the purpose of building muscle mass, you will need to eat anywhere from 3,500 to over 5000 calories per day. Keep in mind that you need to make sure your food is of high quality as well. You need to pay attention to the nutrition values of what you eat in order to gain plenty of minerals and vitamins. The number of calories sounds like a lot, but even on a vegan diet, you can reach those numbers by eating around six meals a day. This is where discipline comes in because you need to have meals prepared every two to three hours. In addition, you need to balance all the fats, carbohydrates, and protein for each meal and perhaps also add some nutritional supplements to compensate for any deficiencies.

Once you have the basics of your nutrition down, you need to focus on training. Again, consistency is what matters. Work smart, not hard. You mustn't skip any workouts just because you feel like you don't have time or you aren't in the mood. Think about your goals, find time and head to the gym. Furthermore, when you're at the gym, you need to give it all you have. You need to train all your muscle groups every week. Do not ignore any of them, no matter how much you hate certain exercises. For instance, many bodybuilders hate the infamous "leg day" because it leaves their legs so tired that they can barely walk up the stairs. It may feel bad in the beginning, but if you ignore such a muscle group you will end up with an uneven look. Your upper body will appear disproportionate when compared to the lower body.

No matter which muscle group you train, and which exercises you choose to do, you should aim to complete three to five sets for each. In between these sets you should also take short rest periods of half a minute to a minute. If you're lifting heavy weights, you can rest up to two minutes instead, especially when training larger muscle groups. Furthermore, when you move from one muscle group to another, you should take a longer break, up to five minutes. Your entire workout should last up to an hour, plus around ten minutes which you take to warm up before getting started.

Preventing Injury

Whether you're a trained athlete or a complete beginner who has never left the office, preventing injury is vital, literally. Whenever you train hard, your body suffers, whether it's from straining your muscles and ligaments to their limit or from nutritional imbalances. Many injuries occur due to not maintaining a correct form when lifting weights, or from pushing the muscles beyond their limit when they're already too fatigued to carry on. Some injuries also occur during the resting period because of an inadequate diet that doesn't supply the body with enough protein, iron, healthy fats and other rich nutrients that are essential for the healing process. Fortunately, it is fairly easy to get the most vitamins, minerals, and protein from a healthy vegan diet. With that being said, here's what you should do to prevent injuries:

1. Being vegan: You've already taken this step, so you have eliminated some potential injuries that may occur from having a meat and dairy focused

diet. Vegetables, fruit, and plants, in general, are much easier to digest and your body will absorb nutrients from them at a much faster pace. Meat is fairly difficult and slow to digest. Therefore your recovery would be slower if you are extracting most of your nutrients from meat. By consuming most of your protein and other vital nutrients from a plant-based diet, your body will recover in time for the next workout. Lifting weights while still recovering can easily cause injuries.

2. Omega 3: This fatty acid is a wonderful nutrient that is healthy for many reasons. In this case, bodybuilders take supplements containing Omega 3 or eat a lot of fish like salmon, because it helps reduce inflammation. Inflammation is one of the most common issues you will encounter because when you're lifting weights. You're essentially tearing your muscles. Therefore they will inflame. Fortunately, you don't have to eat fish to gain this nutrient because it is also found in various seeds and nuts, like walnuts and flaxseed. In addition, you can take it as a supplement made from algae.

3. Turmeric and ginger: As mentioned, inflammation is an issue, so take advantage of everything that

fights it. Spice your diet with ginger and turmeric because both of these ingredients contain compounds that reduce muscle swelling and joint pain.

4. Strengthen your bones: Having healthy and strong bones is crucial when lifting heavy weights. Prevent a number of painful accidents by making sure to consume enough calcium, magnesium and vitamin D. Contrary to popular belief, you don't need to eat dairy products for these vital compounds. All you need to do is eat a lot of green vegetables, nuts and any variety of seeds. Get bonus points to your bone strength by also eating potassium-rich foods like bananas and coconuts.

5. Collagen: This is a powerful ingredient that mustn't be ignored. Many injuries occur because of sensitive ligaments and tendons that aren't flexible enough. When lifting weights you need to make sure that your body can withstand the pressure of lifting a lot of weight. Collagen is what keeps both your tendons and ligaments healthy and flexible. Fortunately, collagen can be found in fruits like strawberries, oranges, lemons

and in any dark leafy vegetables. As a bonus, you will also get a healthy dose of vitamin C, which is important for your bones and ligaments.

6. Drink water: The importance of water cannot be stressed enough. Bodybuilders need to stay hydrated constantly otherwise their joints and muscle tissue will suffer more than they need to.

Bodybuilding doesn't have to be painful if you learn the basics and take one step at a time. It all boils down to having proper nutrition and doing the exercises correctly without overtraining.

What to Expect in the First Few Weeks of Bodybuilding as a Vegan

Making such a dramatic change in your lifestyle, both by going vegan and getting started with bodybuilding comes with a set of challenges. Some of these need to be addressed in the beginning by making various corrections in your diet and exercise program. If you encounter any of the issues we are going to discuss in this section, don't panic and don't allow frustration to ruin your dedication and motivation. With that in mind, here's what you will probably experience in the first few weeks of bodybuilding as a vegan and what you can do about it:

1. Losing weight: As discussed earlier, plant-based diets are nutritious but they don't pack as many calories are your typical modern diet that also includes animal products. This fact alone may lead to weight loss in the first few weeks of making the switch to being vegan. Naturally, this isn't necessarily a challenge or a problem if one of your goals is to also lose weight, not just gain muscle. However, if you aren't overweight and you're looking to increase in mass, this weight loss becomes a serious issue. Fortunately, you can easily adjust your diet to prevent yourself from losing weight. What you should always do no matter what your goals are, is count your calories. Discipline yourself to keep a little logbook with your caloric intake to make sure your body gets enough fuel, or that it doesn't get too much of it. By keeping track, you will know whether you are in a caloric deficit or not. If you are, all you need to do is consume richer foods like any type of nuts, seeds and grains, as well as olives, oils and any variety of nut butters. A simple correction can easily get you back on track.

2. Gaining weight: As a vegan, gaining weight can still be a problem. Plant-based diets don't

automatically translate to being skinny. Plenty of vegans are overweight because there are many vegetables and protein-rich foods that are very high in calories, like those mentioned above. So make sure you inform yourself about your calorie intake and know how many calories there are in everything you eat. Maintaining a basic log will help you keep track of your calories and keep yourself in check.

3. Hunger: Many new vegans complain about always feeling hungry. This could be an issue especially if you used to eat meat and plenty of rich dairy products on a daily basis. This is only normal when making the switch from such a diet because meat and dairy products are very filling due to the protein and fats. However, you can solve this problem by consuming vegan foods that are rich in the same compounds. Protein and fat are filling and can be found in tofu, nuts, seeds and so on. You can also increase your fiber intake because it is also filling. All you need to do is eat more whole grains.

4. Feeling bloated: If you're bloating in the first few weeks it means you need to make another

adjustment to your diet. This issue can be caused either by consuming too much protein or too much fiber, or both! This is especially the case if you suddenly start consuming more fiber and protein than you used to. However, you can easily fight this problem by hydrating yourself. Drink as much pure water as you can throughout the day. You might not feel thirsty, but your diet and your workout routine demand a lot of water. In addition, you could increase your protein consumption gradually so that you give your body a chance to adapt.

5. Not enough protein: If you feel you aren't getting enough protein from your diet you need to start eating more protein-rich foods, like tofu, various beans, and soy curls. If you don't like some of these options, you can always opt for protein supplements. Whatever you choose, make sure to take the carbs into account because protein rarely comes on its own.

6. Eating out: In the beginning, you might be struggling to decide where to eat out. You look at the restaurants in your area and you barely find any specializing in vegan food or you simply

don't like what they have on offer. In this you need to broaden your search. Nowadays, there are many options and most restaurants, pizza places included, have vegan options on their menus. However, if you live in a smaller town, you should still go out because eating out is more about socializing with friends and family than the dining experience itself. So, go out even if you have to grab a boring salad. You can enjoy the company of your friends and then eat something else later when you're on your own at home.

Being a vegan as well as a bodybuilder means adopting a new lifestyle. This isn't about a diet or a sport, but about a way of life, and adapting your body as well as your mind will take a few weeks or even a few months. So, give yourself enough time. Make the changes gradually and be patient with yourself. Soon enough, you will embrace the new lifestyle, or it will embrace you in fact.

Top Transitioning Tips

Switching to a vegan diet can be shocking and even overwhelming, physically, mentally and even emotionally. This statement might sound drastic, but the reality is that changing your lifestyle completely is a drastic change. That is why you need to be knowledgeable about what you're doing. Otherwise, you will give into frustration. Instead of thinking about this change as a daunting task with many unknowns, you should look at it as unlocking a new way of life that comes with a variety of new tastes, smells, and experiences.

Prepare yourself for the new transition and make it as enjoyable as possible by following a few simple tips:

1. Open up to new options: Far too many people are closed-minded when it comes to veganism because our dietary needs are never properly explained. The government doesn't take many steps in educating the population on how to eat healthily and what each ingredient does to the human body. Only in the past few years have people been starting to open up to the idea of giving up on animal products. So open yourself to the many new options you have at your disposal. There are thousands of new recipes for you to try, dozens of new food items you never even thought of tasting, and many ways of cooking. You can gain all the nutrients you need from a vegan diet, while also having fun. Veganism isn't all about

eating boiled broccoli all day and lacking nutrients.

2. Educate yourself: As a free individual, it is your duty to inform yourself about what you consume. After all, you are what you eat. So read up on where your food comes from and what it contains. Don't just eat something because someone tells you it's good for you. Read about nutrition, vitamins and minerals, and about everything that your food contains. Only this way can you make educated decisions on what to eat every day to stay healthy and fit.

3. Stay motivated: You may have started out excited and motivated because veganism and bodybuilding are both something new to you, however, this motivation can easily fade away if you aren't careful. Motivation is important and it will keep you on track with your goals. One of the ways to guarantee that you stay motivated is taking note of whatever made you start on this path in the first place. Memorize it, write it down in a diary, do anything you need to do to remember why you went vegan. This way whenever you feel like giving up, or you have a

moment of weakness, you can take yourself back to the reason why you started everything.

4. Invest in your kitchen: Make your diet as fun and diverse as possible by having everything you need to cook in a multitude of ways. Learn how to make soups and shakes, use a dehydrator and an air fryer. There are so many cool gadgets out there that can cook your food in so many ways without removing all the juicy nutrients. An added bonus to this is the fact that you don't even need to know how to cook in order to make something tasty.

5. Support: Going through change is difficult, but it is far easier if you have someone who can offer you support during your journey. Join a group of vegans on social media and share recipes, talk about your daily challenges and what can be done to improve your diet. Get a fellow vegan training partner and exercise together. Use any channel available to you to connect with people who feel and think the same way you do. This will help you clear your doubts and get over moments of frustration.

As mentioned several times throughout this book, going vegan is a lifestyle, just like bodybuilding.

Therefore, you need to build new habits. You need to rewrite nearly your entire behavior when it comes to food, and new habits don't settle overnight. Be patient with yourself, stay positive, and don't be afraid to ask for some support when you're feeling down.

Summary

Going vegan and getting started with bodybuilding are both two major lifestyle choices that can have nothing but positive impacts on your life if you are knowledgeable enough. That is why in this long chapter we have taken the time to discuss all the basics related to both veganism as well as bodybuilding. You learned what being a vegan really means and that it isn't just about a certain type of diet. You explored all the advantages, as well as the disadvantages of being a vegan and what you can do to overcome all the common challenges you will encounter along with your transition.

In addition, we have discussed the topic of bodybuilding and what it entails. Remember that this sport isn't just about exercising and growing muscles. Again, it is a lifestyle. It changes you mentally and physically for the better. However, it can also overwhelm you if you aren't careful. So make sure to take everything in moderation and pay attention to how you exercise and eat, especially in the first few months.

Furthermore, remember to set a number of goals that will motivate you to stay on track. When making such huge changes in your life, it is easy to fall victim to temptation and go back to your old ways as the excitement fades. Consistency is key when it comes to both bodybuilding and veganism. Stay determined, motivated, and work on yourself one step at a time. There are no miraculous changes that happen overnight, but if you stick with the program, you will change for the better, guaranteed.

CHAPTER 2

Fail-Proof Strategies to ELIMINATE the Most Common Excuses People Have and Defeat Limiting Beliefs So that YOU Can Get Results Fast!

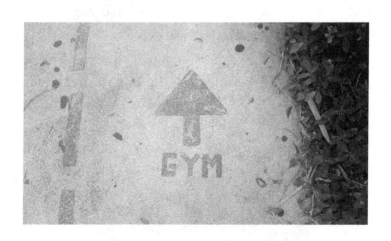

If you are new to bodybuilding or veganism, this chapter will give you answers on how to keep the right mindset and stay motivated. In today's world of fast living, fast transportation, fast food, fast jobs, fast everything, it is almost impossible to stay true to your goals and successfully achieve them. Many people give up whenever they try to change their lifestyle. It is really not easy to go from comfortable, known, and easy to something that is completely new, requires learning; giving up on old habits and strong willpower. There will always be temptations around us and although it seems easy to just give up and indulge in them, think twice, is it really worth it? There is no magic pill that will make the transition for new vegans, bodybuilders or both any easier, but there are some tips and tricks you could learn and they will help you to keep going and achieve the healthy lifestyle you've always desired.

How to Stay Motivated With the Vegan Lifestyle

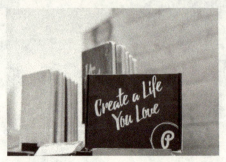

Fail-Proof Strategies to ELIMINATE the Most Common Excuses

The world we are living in, especially the Western world is bombarding us with the information that an animal-based diet is the only way you will get high-quality proteins. There are thousands of fast food joints, snacks, and even restaurants that offer food based on animal products and the options for vegans are sparse. Family and friend dinner parties, even with the best wishes to accommodate everyone, often overlook that one person who's based his diet only on plants, making us feel awkward unintentionally. It is challenging to stay true to yourself and your plant-based diet and sometimes it even feels like the whole world is against you. Do not let feelings and situations like these influence you and make you quit your newly adopted lifestyle that can only lead to long term health and overall wellness. There are small but important things you could do to keep yourself motivated:

1. Remember the reason why you decided in the first place to change your lifestyle to veganism. Be it your moral reasons or health reasons, they are strong enough to get you going. Remind yourself often why it is important to you to achieve the set goals and when it gets difficult, remind yourself how strong the motivation was when you were at the beginning. The feelings of goodness and wellbeing will overflow you, just like in the

beginning of your decision to change your diet, and the motivation will come back.

2. Veganism is not a diet but a lifestyle. People who try plant-based food just because it's the trend will often fail, as they have no good reason or motivation, to begin with. Veganism is a healthy lifestyle and if your motivation is to improve yourself as a whole being—not just your body but your mind too—you will never have problems with a lack of motivation. Keeping the right mindset is very important.

3. Remember the ethical reasons. As said before, veganism is not just a diet. It involves changing your whole life, moral choices too. Think about the way animals are treated when they are considered to be nothing more than a source of food. It extends even to entertainment, as many animals are engaged and abused just for the purpose of our own amusement. Be compassionate towards animals, we share the planet with them; we are not their superior but equals. Being vegan also means thinking about the environment and what we do to our own planet. If you step into the plant-based diet with changed

ethics and moral views, possibilities for keeping the motivation up are never-ending.

4. Keep yourself motivated by watching documentaries. They are a great way of keeping yourself educated and up to date with the new scientific research, but also they will give you insight into how the human modern way of life influences his health, his surroundings and how it hurts the most those who cannot defend themselves. Some movies you should definitely watch include *Vegucated, Food Inc., Food Matters,* and *Earthlings*. These are just examples. With research, you can find a plethora of documentaries that will keep you motivated. Some are free to watch online, some are available on platforms like Netflix or Amazon Prime Video.

5. Read a book! Just like movies, books are an excellent source of information. They can either teach us new information about the life we choose to lead or capture us in their own, unique world that will teach us to appreciate our surroundings and environment. There are even many famous people who wrote their life stories of how a vegan diet helped them overcome their troubles. They

are there to educate, offer support and as a morale boost. Some of the recommended books are *The China Study, Veganomicon, How Not to Die, Animal Liberation, Mad Cowboy* and so many more. In addition to books, you can keep yourself updated by reading relevant vegan articles and blog posts. There are many, many vegan bloggers who offer not just yummy recipes, but also their stories of how life-changing a plant-based diet is, and those will keep you motivated.

How to Stay Motivated with Bodybuilding

Similar to a vegan lifestyle, bodybuilding may require some additional motivation for you to stay on track and achieve your health goals. This is simply because exercise takes time, and there are days when we all would spend our precious time doing something else. Of course, indulging sometimes in relaxation or some other hobbies will do you no harm, but bodybuilding is about developing discipline and keeping to a routine. Sometimes it is hard, and some people simply are not cut out for strict discipline. But there is a way to learn to love it and create a habit of your new, bodybuilding lifestyle.

1. One great way to stay motivated is to often think of the prize, not the process. Keep your goal in

your mind at all times, visualize what you want to achieve and it will get easier to make yourself go to the gym. For some people, the struggle starts with just the thought of the gym, as the pain and effort are more real to them than the goal they are striving to achieve. The trick is to shift your focus from the process of exercise to the end goal. One way to help you visualize what you want to look like is a simple online search for the images of people who inspire you. You need to create the habit of valuing the end prize more than the process of exercising itself. When your end goal is visualized in complete clarity in your mind, you will have no trouble enduring and you will never miss a work-out session.

2. Once you visualize your perfect body, envision work-out sessions as steps that you need to take and that will lead you closer to your perfect self. Each step taken is one step closer to your goal. Each step missed, is you going backward, going away from your goal. Do not miss a work-out, if you need to reschedule it do so, but do not completely miss it out. Allowing your body to relax and indulge in everyday routines of your previous life is a perfect way to lose motivation.

Create a program and stick to it as it will help you conquer new steps each day.

3. Routine is good as it will keep you going and create a habit, and we all know how difficult it is to get rid of habits. However, if you are stagnating and not gaining muscle mass at the speed you desired, simply change the routine. Maybe some other plan and program is better suited for you, and there is nothing wrong with changing it. After all, it keeps the boredom away. Changing the routine is not the same as breaking it completely. Try to stick to the same hours and same gym if possible, but change the exercises you are doing instead. Shift focus from one muscle group to another and see the results of the new routine plan. If you are not satisfied, it's easy to go back to what gave you the best results, or even try a third program. Experiment until you find one that will give you the best results.

4. Pre-workouts are important. It's enough to let thirty minutes pass after you take a powerful pre-workout supplement to feel its effects. This will prepare you not just physically but mentally too. Pre-workout gives you mental stimulation to

continue, lifts your mood and boosts your confidence in what you are doing. Pre-workouts do not have to be expensive! You are just a click away from amazing recipes for homemade pre-workout supplements. We will discuss this topic more in Chapter 3.

5. Personal motivation. We all have that one reason why we want to change our lifestyle and commit ourselves to bodybuilding. It can be anything from health, looks, proving someone wrong, getting that girl… It doesn't matter. Remember what gave you the first boost and motivated you in the first place. Take the satisfaction from visualizing how others will react when they see you at your best! Working out boosts confidence. Imagine all the things you could achieve by looking awesome, feeling healthy and being strong.

6. Sometimes, motivation comes from the simplest things around us. Music, as one example, can be a great mood-lifting medium. With elevated mood comes motivation. Also, who doesn't like working out with a powerful beat giving the rhythm for exercises? The benefits of music on the human mind and body are researched extensively. If you

are interested, find the reading material on the topic, and find your own beat that will best suit your needs.

7. Finally, take a week without training! To fully recover the body after a long-term workout, a pause is needed. It will not only allow you to keep getting better gains, but it will also give you time for yourself which you will spend not thinking about the gym. Soon enough, you will realize you miss the routine of exercising and you will have an increased desire to go back and hit the gym as soon as possible. Keep in mind that one week is enough for your body to undergo full systemic recovery, and the more you delay in returning to the gym, the harder it will be to go back.

Apps to Help You Stay Motivated

Who can imagine life without smartphones these days? They are great helpers in our day-to-day lives and in planning our business. We always have them, if not in our hands then somewhere nearby. The industry of app development has gone beyond what we thought possible just ten years ago. Apps are amazing in helping us overcome daily challenges and they can be amazing in helping us stay motivated and healthy. Here are some great apps you could use but remember, there is no need to have them all. Choose the one that will suit your needs the best. This list is just a guide that will help you visualize what is out there in the market, feel free to experiment with new apps.

1. Nike Training Club: this one is a Nike training app and it is free. This app allows you to choose your goal such as sculpting, toning, strength, and it will select the best workout program based on what you are trying to achieve.

2. MyFitnessPal: is a simple calorie counter in the form of an app. It will keep track of the food you take in on a daily basis. You will be allowed to set caloric goals and input details about your exercises. The app will give you accurate readings of how your diet progresses from day to day.

3. Fit Radio: We already mentioned that music could be a great factor when it comes to workout. Fit Radio will introduce musical workout experience with real famous DJs from all over the world. But it's more than just another music app. It also gives you audio guides for workouts as "cardio coach" will cheer you on. To discover everything that this

app has to offer, you might need to use the option of premium subscription, but the app itself is free.

4. FitBit: the perfect app for the kind of person that needs to track everything. The app allows you to map out your running, hiking or cycling routes. It has a calorie tracker and is amazing with its graphical representation of your activities that will keep you well informed and motivated to go on.

5. Workout Hero: An app that allows you to log your daily workout, monitor your records and even share them with friends using Facebook, Twitter or email. It has a database complete with different recipes depending on what diet you are following, workout and food alarms, checklists, videos, books... Seems like it can do just about anything! However, it is an app developed specifically for Apple devices and it won't work on the Android operating system.

6. Fitocracy: is an app that will make your workout even more fun, shaping it as a game. It will give you points for achieving daily goals, it will send you on fitness quests with which you will be able to earn points and unlock new features. This app is

perfect for those who won't give up their gaming lifestyle.

7. Virtual Runner: is another app that makes the workout fun. This one focuses only on running as it will take you to virtual places of famous races that you can enjoy while on a treadmill. To keep it all competitive, the app will allow you to submit your times for each finished race and it will even reward you with medals for amazing scores.

8. Zombies, Run: an app that will keep you motivated to run for sure! Headphones are a must for this app as it will allow you to hear zombies coming after you, and if you let your imagination go wild, you will get a much-needed morale boost.

9. Happy Cow: this app is perfect for vegan travelers as it acts as a guide for vegan food around the world. It covers 183 countries with helpful information about the restaurants, markets, supermarkets and more. Through this app, you can even contribute with your own newly discovered restaurants, photos or reviews of restaurants that are already in the database.

10. Meetup: This app is all about making it easy to meet people with the same goals, hobbies, and

lifestyles as you. It is not specifically meant to be used just by vegans, or just by bodybuilders, but you can find a community to join, even meet up in person, share ideas, stories and experiences that will boost your motivation. And after all, there are never enough like-minded people in our lives, why not make some new friends? Simply search for vegan bodybuilder groups in your area, and if one doesn't exist, start your own group!

Finding a Workout Partner

While some people enjoy working out alone, as it gives them peace to focus better, others enjoy the company and a little bit of healthy competition a companion brings. Having a workout partner may lift your mood, boost your morale and make exercising an enjoyable effort, not just an obligation. Your workout buddy can be anyone, friend, partner or a family member, as long as it's a person who understands your new lifestyle and fully supports you in it. You do not want someone who will throw negative comments at you, lowering your enthusiasm and draining your energy. Choose your gym partner wisely as the benefits it can bring to your workout routine are amazing.

Fail-Proof Strategies to ELIMINATE the Most Common Excuses

1. Your workouts will be fun if you compare it with someone. Gyms can often be boring places, bring your friends with you and add some good banter and laughter to your workout session. Keep in mind not to overdo it as it can slow you down and distract your focus. Moderate amounts of laughter can only boost your morale and help you reach your goals easier, in a more fun way.

2. Another aspect of exercise is healthy competition. While you and your buddy are keeping fit, you can always introduce little competitive games in your routine that will make your gym time fun. See who can lift more or who can run longer. Make sure your friend is at the same fitness level as you are before competing, as too big of a difference may result in injuries. Also, keep in mind it's all for fun and games and do not push yourself enough to suffer an injury.

3. Having a workout buddy is an excellent way of keeping the routine. Even after a stressful day, when you are not really in the mood for a gym, you will have a partner who will push you, motivate you and give you the much-needed boost to continue going. Discipline is one of the most

important factors in fitness, being regular will only improve your stamina and strength, and having a friendly face on the days when you are just not in the mood, will keep you going.

4. Share the gym expenses with your friends. Sometimes, you can be short on money because of unpredictable expenses and sharing gym time with a friend is a good way to save your funds. Instead of paying for a personal trainer just for you, why not share the expense with a friend? Again, to benefit from a personal trainer equally, it is best if both of you are at the same level of fitness. The trainer's focus won't be divided into two, instead, you will both get equal attention as your needs are the same.

5. While having a friend in the gym with you, the risk of injury is lower. The friend will be there to help you with the gym equipment, or with a word of advice and warning not to overwork yourself. A friend can monitor the position of your body and correct it when it is needed according to the exercise you are doing. Don't forget to return the favor, your friend will only appreciate it.

6. If you are a beginner, and not in great shape, you might feel the awkwardness of going to the gym for the first time, alone. Having a friend with you will help you disperse any fears about the workout you might have. Slowly, your confidence will grow, and you might lose the need for a workout partner, but you will always understand others who might feel awkward exercising alone. For absolute beginners, the best is to have a friend who is on a higher level of fitness, and also patient enough to devote time in showing you around the gym and how to properly use the equipment.

7. Your friends in fitness can only be your asset. Studies have shown that to maintain a certain lifestyle, one must surround himself with like-minded people. They will be your support, motivation, trainers, and partners; people who understand you and who are going through the same thing as you are. They share the same interests with you and friendship will come easy between you. Workout in groups can also be useful. Mixed male and female workout groups also bring their own types of benefits. Experiment and see if a workout partner is a good idea for you that will help you reach your goal.

Exercise Equals Happiness

There are numerous studies to confirm the thesis that exercise makes us feel happier. From our own experience, we can conclude that the simple moving of our body makes us feel better. The constant desire to move and spend energy in one way or another is our primal need. No wonder all cultures in the world affiliate dancing with the moments of happiness. Dancing is just one way of movement, and it sparks joy in people all over the world. Be it just simple clubbing, ritual dancing of various religions, folk dances from around the world or theater dancing. Moving is what we were born to do and what is exercise if not perpetual state of moving one's body?! You do not need to perform complex dance positions in order to feel the benefits of moving, a simple walk, jogging or weight lifting will do. Moving is one of only a few actions that have long-lasting beneficial effects on our brain. In order to feel good, you can eat a chocolate bar and feel instant happiness, but it will be short-lasting and it will have a negative side effect of putting weight on your body. This is the same for alcohol consumption, even though it has the ability to make you feel good for a night, tomorrow you will likely have a hangover and feel bad. Moving or exercise is the only way of having a positive chemical effect on your brain that will lift your mood and make you happier, as well as having the long-lasting effect of making you fit.

A study done at Stanford University showed that only 20 minutes of exercise is enough to keep a person happy for 12 hours. (Denny & Steiner, 2009). So next time you feel sad, not motivated enough, spare some time and allow yourself 20 minutes of workout session to lift your mood and boost your morale.

How exactly does exercise lift our mood? The simple answer is endorphins. They are hormones produced by our central nervous system and the pituitary gland. The main job of endorphins is to inhibit the transmission of pain signals. However, they also produce a feeling of euphoria. It is this feeling that instantly makes us happy, and since it's a completely natural process that occurs within us, it has no negative impact on any segment of our body.

Endorphins are not the only hormone that is produced while exercising and it is not the only one that makes us happy. Other chemicals our bodies produce are serotonin, norepinephrine, BDNF, and dopamine. All of these chemicals have a huge positive impact on our minds. Even depression is treated with the inclusion of body activity as it is a natural way of healing both mind and body.

There is another very interesting study done on both Oxford and Yale and it shows that exercise makes people happier than money. Physical activity has such a great impact on mental health, greater than economic status! The study even gives results on which sports activities have the most benefits for the mind. While most of them involved in team sports, gym and weight lifting took the high spot as a sport that had the greatest impact on overall happiness (Chekroud, Gueorguieva, Zheutlin, Paulus, Krumholz, Krystal, et al., 2018).

Why Bodybuilders Must Master Meditation

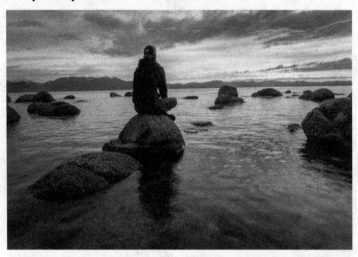

Recent studies performed by the American Heart Association showed that meditation is greatly linked with the prevention of inflammatory conditions, heart disease, and stroke. But that is not all, the same research came to the conclusion that meditation helps with faster physical recovery, especially after stressful situations and injuries (Levine et al., 2017). But how is this important for bodybuilders? Athletes, in general, can greatly benefit from faster physical recoveries and bodybuilders are among them. Besides physical benefits, meditation will also help us better focus on exercises we are doing which will result in higher intensity training. Meditation also helps bodybuilders to cope with pain better as they are putting stress on their muscles. Meditation reduces stress and anxiety which is important for some people, especially those who love to join competitions. Other physical benefits of meditation include hormone balance which leads to a stable, well-balanced organism. Meditation also helps with sleep, making it easier, deeper and regular. Sleep is important for bodybuilders as it is the time our bodies are recovering fastest.

Meditation also leads to molecular changes in our body that are extremely beneficial for bodybuilders. The levels of pro-inflammatory genes are reduced and the physical recovery is faster. Even inexperienced subjects can greatly benefit from practicing meditation.

If you wonder if you really must sit in an uncomfortable position while chanting mantras in unknown languages to achieve meditation, the answer is no. Leave that to the hippies who like exotic stuff. For meditation to have its beneficial effect on the human body, it is enough to relax in any position that suits you and focus your mind on the present while being fully aware of your thoughts. However, it is not beneficial to judge yourself, so try as best as you can to be objective towards your own body. Do not worry about the future or the past while meditating. It is really important to be aware of the present and where you are at a given moment. After a while of practicing meditation, you will gain the ability to transcend your thoughts and you will become more clearly aware of what are you doing, why are you doing it and how to achieve your goals. The exercising won't be just exercising, but a conscious effort that leads to healthier change. Eating plant-based food won't be just eating, but an important part of your own choices and decisions you made in order to better yourself. Your purpose will become clear to you and your actions will reflect it more naturally. Meditation is regarded as something that is supposed to calm you, but after practicing it for a certain time period, you will notice your passion for achieving your goals is returning, and you will find new will in you that will keep you going forward.

Vanquishing Common Excuses For Not Going To The Gym

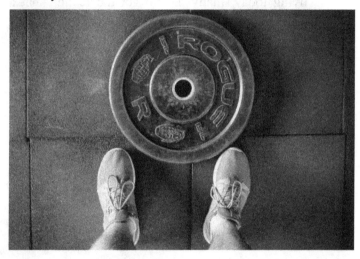

Getting started with the gym can often be the most difficult part of bodybuilding for beginners. Various studies showed that surprisingly high numbers of people in the world are members of the gym. However, the majority of them don't use their membership at all. Maybe you can recognize yourself among them. Yes, going to the gym is an obligation, but in the previous sections we saw it could be fun, it is beneficial to your body and mind, it has no negative impact on a person's life whatsoever. The myriad of people who avoid going to the gym even with having the membership have exactly the same excuses. Some of the most common excuses are complete nonsense! Let's see why:

1. "I don't have time": because of the fast way of living today, many people get the feeling that a day doesn't have enough hours, and an hour spent in the gym is a wasted hour. However, workouts help you increase your productivity and with it you will gain much needed time, not lose it. Also, working out during the workday helps us to clear our minds, and boost our happiness and health. Studies have shown that not only the productivity increase in people who exercise during weekdays but also they need fewer sick days as they are generally healthier!

2. "I'm too tired": Yes, the majority of people have busy lives that won't allow them to exercise at any other time except after work when they already spent most of their energy. But we already said that after work exercise could lift your stress off your shoulders and prepare your body for meaningful rest. In time, your energy levels will increase and you won't feel tired after a stressful day at work.

3. "I am shy because I don't know what I am doing": Many people quit their gym membership because they either feel out of place there, or they are intimidated by "regulars" who are at much higher fitness level then they are, and they feel shy for not knowing even the basics. However, this is no excuse at all. Nobody was born in the gym, and no one knew what to do from the start. Even that guy in the middle of the gym who looks like he was cut off the mountainside was once new and had to learn his moves. Besides, the chances are that you are not the only new person in the gym that is much greater than you think. After all, this is exactly why gyms offer trainers, beginner programs and even discounts for new people. Their job is to help you learn and train you.

4. "Other people stare at me". This is a basic misconception about the gym. People do not have much interest in you, no matter how important you think you are. They are all focused on what they are doing and how they are doing their own techniques as exercising is not just lifting weights. People need to be careful not to injure themselves, and to engage the right group of muscles. You will also notice many bodybuilders have headphones

on as the music helps them isolate themselves and focus better at what they are doing, so their gaze won't wander over at the newbie like yourself. If someone does throw a glance at you, it might be that he wants to make a new friend, help you perform your exercise better, congratulate you on a good job! People at the gym share common interests and are often the easiest people you will make friends with.

Dispel Toxic Beliefs on Vegan Bodybuilding

Even the people who are long term vegans have trouble with doubts about their diet, and the world around us is not making it easy with its misconceptions that we need meat in order to be strong and big. This misconception is especially strong among athletes and particularly bodybuilders. To keep being not just big and strong, but healthy as well, vegan bodybuilding is simply the best choice. Whether you are just a beginner in a plant-based diet or an experienced member of the vegan community, you too have certainly met people who will try to persuade you why meat is necessary for the human body. However, with consuming meat, you are more likely to accelerate cancer growth and to age much faster. Meat is simply high in fat and filled with contaminants whether from the environment or from deliberate injection from people who grow animals for food. Sure, it is easier to bulk up while eating meat, but it does come with a cost, as your hormone production will change and your testosterone levels will grow. Bodybuilders who eat meat get sick more often and have digestive problems when compared to vegans. Here are some of the most usual misconceptions about a vegan diet and bodybuilding, and in this part of the chapter, we will try to debunk them.

1. People need a lot of animal protein for quick recovery after working out. This myth is simply not true as it is known that only 10% of daily caloric intake needs to be from protein in order for athletes muscle to recover. A plant-based diet can easily meet these needs plus it will provide you with fiber and phytonutrients that meat doesn't contain. However, what really matters when it comes to protein is its absorption rate. Eating large quantities of protein means nothing if it's not absorbed by your body. Many meat-eaters will eat too much animal-based proteins that will end up stored in their body as fat. However, the fiber in plants helps vegans digest proteins properly, speeding up their absorption.

2. Animal protein is superior to plant protein. This misconception is so common, that people refer to animal protein as "quality" protein. However, plant-based protein is equally good for bodybuilders and some vegetables, fruits, nuts, and seeds contain even more protein than meat. There are numerous recipes of plant-based protein bars, salads and shakes a bodybuilder can use to fuel himself. Chickpeas, quinoa, raw nuts, hemp seeds and many, many more are just some of the examples of excellent plant-based protein sources that will satisfy your daily needs.

3. A vegan diet doesn't have enough nutrients. Another common misconception as people tend to believe vegans are weak and sickly looking, but this is far from the truth. Yes, not all vegans are healthy, many of them make simple mistakes with their diet, just like meat-eaters, or vegetarians. Proper nutrition demands knowledge and learning. But plant-based diet has proved to be one of the healthiest diets in the world. It is also common to believe that vegans have to substitute some of the essential nutrients by using supplements. This is mainly thought of as vitamins such as B12, Iron, and Zinc. And yes, some vegans prefer

supplements, but there are plenty of plant-based sources of these substances. Nutritional yeast, spinach, and soy milk are rich in vitamin B12, while beans, raisins and prunes are loaded with iron. For zinc it is recommended to eat lots of legumes, nuts and seeds.

4. Vegans lack energy and strength as they cannot bulk up like meat-eating bodybuilders. Another misconception that it is very popular among bodybuilders. But the sheer number of vegan bodybuilders who are successful in competition and who are winning should be proof enough that this misconception is ridiculous. We will talk more about them in the next section, as they serve as an excellent example of keeping you motivated.

Summary

Staying motivated is an important part of any lifestyle change you are planning to make. Sometimes, people are just too happy to give up the comfort of their previous life is pulling them. However, regrets and disappointments will follow. Being true to yourself and your goals is the best thing you can do to achieve a happy and healthy life. Even though we all have days when we are down, we need to learn how to fight them. In this chapter, you found the weapon and knowledge that will help you conquer those moody days when you ask yourself is it really worth it? But you already know the answer, being healthy and looking good beside it is always worth it. You learned that exercise, especially bodybuilding brings more happiness than even money. It is also extremely healthy. Now you also know you don't have to be alone on your new journey. Find a partner who will help you keep the motivation up and who will also help you achieve your goals. If not a partner, then try one or more of the smartphone apps specially designed to provide you with support. Some of them are even fun and make you forget about all the hard work with simple amusement they offer. Don't forget to train your spirit and mind just as you are training your body. Meditation and clarity of mind will help you in this, but they will also help your body heal faster and grow stronger. Look at the example of some of the famous bodybuilders and their achievements. They are pure images of health and happiness that you can achieve just as easily.

👀 Look! Special Offer Currently Available! 👀

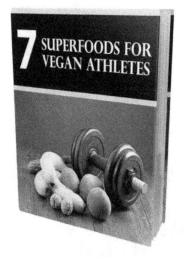

⚠ Warning: Downloads of this book have been limited to 15 FREE Downloads. Then, the price instantly shoots up to $27 ⚠

Hurry! Get Your Copy Now by Clicking the Link Below:

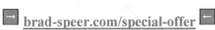

brad-speer.com/special-offer

Here's just a fraction of what you'll discover:

- 7 secret superfoods that you had NO IDEA existed!
- A secret superfood to increase the release of testosterone!
- How these foods can enhance your overall health and build muscle too!

...and so much more!!

Fail-proof Guide to Vegan Bodybuilding and Fitness

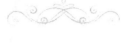

CHAPTER 3

Nutrition Secrets Revealed For Vegan Bodybuilders... Even If You're on a Tight Budget or Pressed for Time

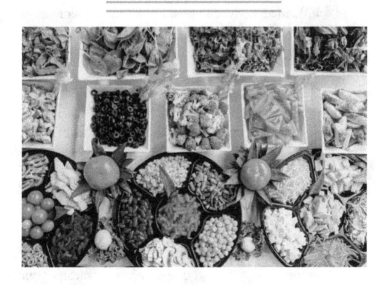

Being a vegan bodybuilder does come with some challenges, but they are all in the area of nutrition. No special vegan plan for exercises exists, and the exercises should remain the same as for any other type of bodybuilders. Training and nutrition are the two most important parts of being a successful bodybuilder and each comes with its own challenges. However, it is the nutrition part that requires special attention if you choose to base your meals on plants. Here is how to overcome some of the biggest nutritional challenges if you are a vegan bodybuilder:

1. Calorie intake for muscle building: Calories are one of the most important factors that will influence body composition. When it comes to bodybuilding, body composition fluctuates on a regular basis, depending on your physique goals and if there are upcoming competitions. Bodybuilders go through phases of losing fat and building muscles over a certain period of time. Both of these phases demand different calorie intake through nutrition. When you are building your muscles and you need to stimulate growth, you will need to significantly increase your calorie intake. This can be challenging even for omnivores. When you are vegan, it means your

plant-based food will have fewer calories, and if you are new to the vegan lifestyle, this can be extremely challenging. However, every challenge can be won, there are plant-based meals that can help you achieve your daily intake of calories, no matter how high. Awesome high-calorie foods for vegans are avocado, nuts, berries, dried fruits, rice, quinoa and legumes. Plan your meals and combine the ingredients in delicious recipes that will help you build strength and stimulate muscle growth.

2. Protein intake challenge: Vegans are limited in the number of food products that will help them take in the desired amount of protein. Strength training demands intake of high amounts of quality proteins as it plays an important role in repairing and rebuilding the muscle tissue. The stress of workout is damaging our muscles, and it is the process of healing that will grow them bigger and stronger. For the healing process, our body needs protein which will optimize the building and recovery of the tissue. Some vegans find it extremely difficult to consume enough proteins as their diet is limited. But it is not impossible. Legumes, pulses, and nuts are high in proteins but

because of their limited choice, some vegans will feel the need to consume vegan-friendly supplements. We will talk more about protein in upcoming parts of the chapter, its role and importance in bodybuilding, and how vegans can fulfill their daily needs without consuming animal products.

3. Challenges in macronutrient balance: Macronutrients are extremely important when it comes to a phase in which you need to lose body fat. It is not as important during the muscle-building phase as calorie intake becomes of greatest importance, but when you are preparing for competition, and when you need to reduce that extra fat, special care is needed. Achieving a balance between fats, proteins, and carbohydrates will give you the best results. We already said proteins are needed for muscle growth. Carbohydrates will be your main source of energy during this phase. Fats are needed as they act as the main factor responsible for the absorption and transportation of nutrients through your body. Macro balancing is important when you are maintaining your muscle size and enhancing physique during this phase of bodybuilding.

4. Deficiencies of micronutrients: We explained what macronutrients are and what their role is. How about micronutrients? They are vitamins, minerals and other trace chemicals our body needs to function properly. In bodybuilding, micronutrients are important as they drive the growth of muscles. They also help with improving your immune system, energy production, bone health, fluid balance and other body factors that influence muscle growth, their health and overall wellness. Vegans find it challenging to consume enough of some vitamins such as B6, B12 and D. Also, iron, calcium, riboflavin and alpha-linolenic acid are usually found in animal-based foods. Because of this, some vegans will need to take supplements to ensure the body is rich enough in micronutrients to function normally, maintain general health and fight off fatigue after training.

To ensure your intake of all the needed nutrients it is important to plan your meals ahead and plan them well. Vegan bodybuilding diet will greatly improve your general health and help you recover after training much faster. However, there are other factors that will influence how well you are performing. Don't forget that sleep is as important as nutrients. It is a phase when our body is resting, but it is also rebuilding. Nutritional challenges you face as a vegan bodybuilder shouldn't be too much of a problem as long as you approach them smartly. Calculate your meals, supplement if you require extra and consult your doctor whenever you feel the need, even if it is just to make sure everything is alright.

What and When to Eat as a Vegan Bodybuilder

It is a popular opinion that as a vegan bodybuilder the choices of food that are able to sustain you and help you grow muscles will be sparse. However, from the experience of some world-renowned athletes, vegan food is usually at the top when it comes to favorite choices. Even omnivorous bodybuilders listed some vegan foods as their top options which not just give them the best results, but also satisfy their nutritional needs. Oats, rice, yams, broccoli and potatoes were listed as top five favorite bodybuilder's foods, no matter what their dietary preference is. This is really encouraging information as it means you won't have to make compromises and you will be able to stick to your plant-based diet. No morals or ethics you might have as a driving force behind your veganism will be endangered. Red meat, fish and eggs were the ingredients that followed, naturally as they are very high in protein. But we already saw that there are great vegan alternatives to intake enough proteins. If you are still confused as to what to eat exactly while training, here is a section that discusses food in detail.

Protein

Let's begin with protein as it is one of the main ingredients every bodybuilder needs in order to grow strong and bulky muscles. In the vegan bodybuilding community, there is something called the "protein pyramid" as there are three main plant-based sources of protein: nuts and seeds, cereals, and legumes.

Earlier, vegans believed that they had to combine at least two of these protein sources in one meal in order to take in enough of it. However, this was recently disproven by various studies, at least when it comes to a simple vegan diet. As a bodybuilder, you might want to continue eating protein from two plant-based sources, or even all three. There are no studies done on vegan bodybuilders yet, and precaution will not hurt you. Ingredients that are an excellent choice of plant-based proteins: tempeh, tofu, oats, lentils, seitan, edamame, chickpeas, quinoa, peas, hempseed, teff, amaranth, and nutritional yeast.

Fat

It often gets a bad reputation as we see it as something unhealthy that will stick to our body and make us gain unwanted weight. However, fat is one of the most essential nutrients for the human body as its role is to transfer another chemical to the various cells in our body. It also helps with the absorption of other nutrients, minerals, and essential chemicals. When we say fat, we often think about meat and its grease. But meat does not contain healthy fats. Instead, it contains trans and unsaturated fats which should be avoided at all costs.

Remember that trans fats are also byproducts of vegetable oils and are added to certain veggie spreads as well as snacks and fried foods. They are the main reason for various inflammations, strokes, heart disease and diabetes. It is a plant-based diet that will provide you with saturated fats. Ingredients such as nuts, seeds, avocados, and plant-based oils are good sources of fat.

There are some fats that are available to vegans in lesser quantities than needed for the normal function of the body, such as Omega-3 DHA and EHA. They are mainly found in fish and other seafood ingredients. A different kind of Omega-3 called ALA is in abundance in the vegan diet. However, the human body needs to convert ALA to DHA/EHA and even though it is capable of it, the conversion itself is not efficient. This is why supplementing Omega-3 is important for vegans, especially bodybuilders. Fortunately, there are products out there on the market that are vegan-friendly since the base for their production is sea algae. Coconut oil is much recommended in the vegan community and it is needed for bodybuilders. However, it is saturated fat and because of it, it needs to be consumed with limitations and care. Saturated fats are easily recognized as they are solid at room temperature. Avoid overusing them as they are another factor that accelerates certain diseases just like trans fats.

Carbohydrates

The first thing your muscles look for when they are in need of energy is your carbohydrate stores. The Dietary Guidelines for Americans recommends that carbohydrates make up 45-60% of daily calorie intake (U.S. Department of Health and Human Services and U.S. Department of Agriculture, 2015). Carbohydrates are broken down in our body into glucose which is then stored in the liver and muscles where it takes the form of glycogen. These glycogen stores are what fuel the body while you work out. Some studies suggest that people on low carb diets are not able to perform as well as people whose intake is higher. However, with carbs we also have to be careful. Your diet needs to be diverse, and the amount of carbs needs to cycle.

When the body gets used to the same diet from day to day, it will adjust, and the desired effect of a diet will not be achieved. Also, processed carbs raise insulin levels. We need insulin to signal our muscles that it is time for them to pull in nutrients. But when we eat carbs all the time, we might begin to suffer from chronically high insulin levels. This means your body will respond to insulin less and the muscles won't pull in needed nutrients and will stop growing. This is how many vegans start gaining fat and find it hard to lose it. This is why carb cycling is a thing when it comes to bodybuilding. And it should look like this: On your priority workout days, you need to boost your carb intake by 25%. On your other workout days, leave your carb intake at the base which you will determine based on how many calories you need to take in. On your rest days, reduce the number of carbs by 25%. This way carbs and total calories will fluctuate, and this will prevent you from gaining fat while bulking up.

Carbs are one of the easiest vegan ingredients as they are everywhere. However, you must understand the difference between the complex carbs which are rich with vitamins and minerals and simple processed carbs which are often called "empty calories" as they have little nutritional value. Complex carbs can be found in black/brown rice, sweet potatoes, lentils, oats, beans, peas, vegetables and many more ingredients. You can indulge in processed carbs on occasion but keep it minimal. They are easily found in pastas and breads.

Amino Acids

Amino acids are building blocks of protein. Bodybuilders need them in order to grow muscles. In total, there are 21 amino acids. However, our body is capable of synthesizing only 12, while the other 9 have to be consumed through food. There are plenty of plant-based foods that contain enough amino acids for vegans to enjoy. However there is one problem with them. The bioavailability of amino acids from plants is lower than from meat and animal products. This means that as vegan, you will have to consume more in order to gain the same amount of amino acids as omnivore bodybuilder. The problem with it is that by eating more, you will consume more calories than your body requires, and they will be stored as fat. By eating varied and well-balanced plant-based foods you will eliminate the danger of not receiving enough amino acids. However, as a bodybuilder, you should think about supplementing them, especially when you are training hard and preparing for the competition.

Timing Your Meals

The timing of meals is very important when it comes to bodybuilding no matter what dietary plan you are following. The common agreement among athletes is that having 6-8 meals will help you grow muscle faster. This means you will have 3 or 4 big meals and 3 to 4 snacks. Eat at intervals of 2 hours and you will not feel hungry if you plan your meals and balance them well. Be prepared and pack your foods for on the go if needed. Freeze extra food as sometimes you will simply have no time for food preparation. When it comes to bodybuilding, it is important to know what and when to eat pre- and post-workout. Timing is extremely important as it can lead to delayed recovery and compromised results if you do not follow the norms. Both pre- and post-workout food will help you build muscle, recover from training, and prepare you for efficient subsequent workouts. When it comes to pre-workout meals, remember that you are allowed to have a full meal 2-4 hours before the session, and if it's a snack, you are allowed to eat it 1-2 hours before a workout. If your aim is to bulk up, do not skip pre-workout food. However, if you are about to have a short cardio training, it might be wiser not to eat before, as food can lead to feeling nausea and stomach cramps. A good pre-workout snack can be a peanut-butter sandwich or soy-yogurt with fruit. It is even more important to fuel your body after a workout session. When you are eating the right amount of certain nutrients after a workout, you are helping your body recover and grow muscle. Have a snack right after your gym session and eat a mixture of protein and carbs. Do not forget that snacks are a part of your daily calorie intake and count them in. You can mix yourself a smoothie using these ingredients:

1 banana, 1 teaspoon of soy yogurt, 1 or 2 teaspoons of vegan-friendly protein supplement, 1 teaspoon of peanut butter and add soya milk to fill up the pint. Instead of banana, you can use any other fruit you might like or even mixed fruits, but don't forget they have calories too, and you shouldn't overdo it. Use fruit like pineapple and papaya as they contain enzymes that will help you absorb protein better.

Lastly, water is very important, and you shouldn't be thinking about leaving the house without it. Take it everywhere with you. Hydrate your body to keep it working properly.

All About Calories

When speaking about nutrition we say calories are a measure for nutritional energy. It is the energy we need for day-to-day life. Your body is burning calories to fuel itself even when you simply walk, talk or breathe. Calories are spent on anything we do in life, as we need fuel to function. When we go to the gym or go running, or do any kind of exercise, we are burning additional calories. However, if we are consuming more calories than our bodies are able to burn, we will gain weight as the body is storing unspent calories for later use. Losing weight is as simple as eating fewer calories than your body burns. Gaining weight is the opposite. You need to consume more calories than your body burns. There is also a third stadium where you consume exactly the same number of calories as your body is spending on a daily basis and you will stagnate. This phase is called maintenance.

It is possible to only eat junk food and lose weight as long as you are burning more calories than you are consuming. However, not all food has the same nutritional value. Fried foods, sugars, and alcohol all have high caloric value but little to no nutritional value. They are poor in macro and micronutrients which our body needs to keep functioning properly. This is why it's not the same when you lose weight eating only fast food, vs when you lose weight by properly balancing your vegan meals. Your goal should always be a healthy lifestyle which will bring good looks.

If you want to lead a healthy life as a vegan bodybuilder, calculating your calories is something that needs to become a routine. The first thing to do is to calculate the number of calories your body requires for maintenance. This specific number is called total daily energy expenditure (TDEE). Calculating TDEE is pretty easy but you need to know the percentage of your body fat. The best way to find out your body fat percentage is to visit a doctor's office. Even though there are scales that can do the calculations for you, they are not as precise.

Now is the time to calculate your lean body mass (LBM) in kilograms. Use your weight and multiply it by (1-fat percentage). Let's say you weigh 80 kg and your body fat is at 15%. Your LBM is calculated: 80x(1-0.15)=68kg.

The next thing you need to do is to estimate your metabolic rate (BMR). Insert your LBM into this formula:

370+(21.6xLBM)=BMR. With the LBM of 62 from the previous example, the mathematics will look like this: 370+(21.6x68)=1838 calories. There is one more way to calculate your BMR and it is widely accepted Harris-Benedict equation. It differs between the sexes as men and women need to have different requirements to power their bodies. Other variables like age, height, and weight need to be put into the equation. The formula for men is (66+(13.7xweight in kg)+(5xheight in cm)-(6.8xage).

For women it is (655+(9.6x weight in kg)+(1.7x height in cm)-(4.7xage).

To calculate properly your TDEE you will need to multiply your BMR by your activity factor. There is a guideline that will help you determine your activity factor and multiply it with your BMR.

Sedentary activity factor (no exercise during the week) BMRx1.1

Lightly active (light exercise from 1 to three days a week) BMRx1.2

Moderately active (3-5 days per week of moderate exercise) BMRx1.35

Very active (hard exercise 6-7 days during a week) BMRx1.45

Extremely active (Very hard exercise + physical job, or exercise two times a day, every day in a week) BMRx1.6-1.8

Now that you know how to calculate your maintenance calories it is easy to adjust them for bulking or cutting. When you are in the bulking phase you need to increase your TDEE by 10%. The extra calories will help you gain around 1-2kg per month if your activity factor stays the same and if you are a man. For women, the extra calories will bring a gain of 0.5 to 1kg per month. Note that both males and females will have higher results if they are new to bodybuilding and the gain can go well over 2kg. If you are cutting you need to reduce your TDEE by 20%. This way you will lose approximately 2-3kg per month and the amount will be the same for both men and women.

There are online calculators that can help you calculate all of the factors you need to determine your TDEE. They will even go so far to calculate your needed deficit or surplus of calories based on your goals. Feel free to try them out to save time and to better focus on your diet and workouts.

Everything You Need to Know About Macros and Micros

Macro is just a short term for macronutrients: the fat, protein and carbs which we covered in the previous segment of the chapter. However, when it comes to calorie counting, it is important to balance your macronutrients. This means that you need to decide precisely how many calories you want to be based on proteins, carbs, and fats. The math is pretty simple as 1 gram of proteins equals 4 calories, 1 gram of carbs equals 4 calories and 1 gram of fat equals 9 calories. Alcohol is sometimes considered macro too as its value per gram is 7 calories. However, it doesn't have any nutritional value and is not recommended for consumption when it comes to bodybuilding. There are many calculators and apps that can help you with balancing your macros but be aware that most of them won't give you the option to calculate the values with alcohol.

The ratios of macronutrients will vary as you change your bodybuilding phases. Your health goals are also important and be sure to adjust macro ratios to cover all your body needs. Remember that counting calories are not the same as tracking your macros. The number of calories you need to intake will not tell you the balance between carbs, proteins, and fats. However, the balance between macros will build up to the desired number of calories. This is why bodybuilders and athletes in general, who only count their calories have fewer results than those who concentrate on the source of the calories. While calorie deficit will make you lose fat, no matter their source, they will not build up your muscles or repair them after the workouts.

When calculating your macros, you need to take several factors into consideration: your weight, your BMI and your activity level. You will also have to adjust your macros depending on what you want to achieve. You will not intake the same number of calories from carbs when you want to lose weight, or maintain muscle mass. The general rule is to lose weight while keeping or increasing muscle mass. To achieve this, your calorie intake has to be sourced with 1 or 1.2 grams of protein per pound of body weight, fat intake needs to be between 0.2 and 0.25 grams per pound of body weight, and the rest of calories you can gain from carbs. Remember that this equation will work only for losing weight and gaining muscle and only if your metabolism and body are healthy. From this starting point, you will be able to adjust the diet depending on how your body reacts to it.

There are many online calculators that will help you count your calories and their sources. With a simple click you can set up your parameters like weight and BMI, you can select the desired program like bulking up, maintenance or lose fat. The calculator will tell you exactly how many calories you need to take and how much protein, carbs, and fat you will use in your daily meals to achieve the desired results. One of the most popular calculators online is Chronometer. It even offers a smartphone app so you can log your details on the go. It will also suggest great vegan recipes that will satisfy your daily caloric needs in the best possible way.

Let's take a closer look at each macronutrient separately and see what their role in our body is and how they influence our bodybuilding goals:

Protein: is a macronutrient essential to bodybuilding as it promotes muscle growth and repair. Vegans often tend to not focus on proteins too much, but when it comes to bodybuilding it's a must! Protein source of macronutrients will provide us with essential amino acids that will repair our muscles and while doing so, they will rebuild them, stronger and bigger. There are various studies that show how protein intake improves muscle gains and increases strength performance. You need to take larger amounts of protein when you are leaning down. This means you will lose less muscle mass during the cutting phase. Protein also makes you feel less hungry because it reduces the levels of hunger hormone ghrelin while increasing the levels of peptide YY, hormones that make you feel full. It also helps with reducing fat by providing thermic effect and during energy restriction. The amount of needed protein for a bodybuilder is an individual thing. It all comes down to what your goal is and at what stage of fitness you are in the given moment. Many bodybuilders agree that it's enough to consume 0.73-1 grams of protein per lbs. per day. However, since the plant-based protein is less anabolic than animal-based protein, feel free to lean towards the higher side of the recommended intake. Our bodies simply don't digest plant-based protein as efficiently, this is due to lack of essential amino acid named leucine. Also, we already mentioned that a higher intake of protein is helpful to maintain or even increase muscle mass while you are in the process of losing weight.

The mathematics come down to this example: a 176-pound vegan bodybuilder would need to eat 176x0.73 or around 128 grams of protein.

Fats: We already mentioned that carbs are amazing for athletes who want to improve their muscle mass and their strength. This is why we prioritize them over the fats, but in general, there is no rule as to how much fat you need as a vegan bodybuilder. Fats will have different effects on different bodies due to essential fatty acids and the person's need for them. Some vegan bodybuilders do well on low-fat diets, others perform better on high-fat diets. You will have to observe your body and see how it responds. But if you want the carbs to influence your bulking up, do prioritize them over fats. However, do not opt for a diet without any fats,as they are essential for your body to work properly. We already talked about the difference between saturated, unsaturated and trans fats. Be careful to balance them well. A bodybuilder generally needs 15-30% of calories to be from fats in order to benefit from it. Whether it will be closer to 15% or 30% depends if you are trying to lose weight, or to bulk up and prepare for competitions.

The math for fats should look like this: If you need to intake 2800 calories per day, you will need 2800x0.15 or 30 =420 or 840 calories that come from fats. Further, because 1 gram of fat contains 9 calories, you will need to intake 47 to 93 grams of fat.

Carbs: are essential for vegan bodybuilders and are not unhealthy in any way. They help us store glycogen which will be used by muscles as fuel thus enhancing our performance. They also play a role in repairing muscle tissue during the bulking phase. There is no need to cut down on carbs as it will only reduce your strength performance as well as the endurance of your muscles, especially when you are cutting down the calories. When you are trying to build your muscles, you will want to keep your carb intake high, but there is no special guideline to tell you how many grams per day are needed. When you are calculating your macros, depending on your goal, do the math for protein and fats, and fill the rest with carbs.

Let's say you are a 176-pound bodybuilder with a need to intake 2800 calories. You decided to consume 150 grams of protein and 70 grams of fat. The end math, in this case, will look like this: 150x4 =600 calories from protein, 60x9= 630 calories from fats. To reach 2800 calories you need to take per day, you will need 2800-(600+630)=1570 calories from carbs. To convert it to grams 1570/4=393 grams.

We mentioned that:

1 gram of protein = 4 calories

1 gram of carbs = 4 calories

1 gram of fat = 9 calories

Use this table when you are converting calories to grams and you will have no problem when macromanaging.

When we are talking about macronutrients we have to mention micronutrients too. It is important not to confuse these two. Micronutrients are vitamins, minerals and other chemicals needed for your body to function properly. Vegans are known to suffer from micronutrient deficits due to bad choices in food. There are supplements, but there is also a way to calculate your micros and get them right just from food. Of course, in some cases supplements are the only choice (Vitamin D and EPA and DHA), but if you want you can micromanage the rest. Many bodybuilders prefer supplements as they are much easier to get and are not that expensive. There is a large number of micronutrients to observe. Vitamins, iron, zinc, calcium are just to name a few and you will need regular visits to a doctor if you want to observe the levels of your micronutrients. Luckily there is no need to do this. Just eat a rich, whole food vegan diet and you will not have to worry if you are getting enough micronutrients.

Supplement those that do not exist in a plant-based diet and you shouldn't have to worry.

How to Plan Your Meals While on a Budget

People often give up from following a purely vegan lifestyle because it can be extremely expensive. If you go to your local store and try to fill your cart with vegan products you will agree that it is really not affordable. However, take a closer look. You will see that the most expensive items on your shopping list are not vegetables and fruits themselves. It's pre-packaged and prepared foods advertised for vegans such as vegan cheese, vegan meat, vegan bacon, or already prepared whole vegan meals. In order to be a vegan and still stay on a budget, you will need to learn how to properly plan your meals and shop accordingly. Here is some advice that will help you with how to do it.

1. Plan your meals in advance and stock up on ingredients. We live in a consumer society and impulse buying is something we all experience. It leads to overspending and often buying ingredients we will not even use. The key to budget shopping is preparation. Sit down at least once a week and plan your meals in detail. Plan each day in a week and prepare a grocery

shopping list. For some items, you can even plan months in advance and stock up. Buying larger quantities is often cheaper and it will cut down your spending. Items such as legumes, nuts and seeds, rice, quinoa, dried fruits, and herbs are long-lasting. If you are missing ideas when you are planning meals for the whole week, use a vegan cookbook and let it be your guide.

2. Use discounts. There are many alternative stores where you could buy your vegan food, it doesn't have to be the one you are used to and that one that's closest to your apartment. Even if you have to walk a bit more to get a good deal or a retail price, it's worth it. Many cities have specialized ethnic grocery stores that you could try as they tend to be cheaper than big well-known supermarket chains. Another great aspect of trying out new stores such as Asian or Middle Eastern is that you will be introduced to new plant-based foods. You can add them to your existing dietary plans as substitutes, or as enrichment to your meals.

3. Don't follow the trends. There are always trends that come and go, but they are often a trap for

your wallet. Trends are always expensive. Stick to the staples, foods you already tried out and are ok with their price and quality. Ingredients such as oatmeal, rice, pasta, lentils, nuts, and seeds should always be on top of your shopping list. Extravaganzas as "new superfoods" are a marketing trick you should avoid.

4. Love your leftovers. Try not to waste food. Leftovers can always be re-packed and frozen for some other day. It will not just help you save food but also preparation time. There will be days when you are in a hurry and you simply have no time to cook. Instead of opting for an unhealthy and expensive vegan snack, you will quickly unfreeze your leftovers and enjoy a healthy meal.

5. Don't fall for the brands. Generic food from your local supermarket may be much cheaper and of the same quality. Usually, this happens because you pay more for the packaging of the big brand food. Generic ones come in simple and cheap packages but will offer the same quality. Read the ingredients carefully and opt for the cheaper version.

6. Carry your own snacks and beverages. When you are going for a hike, to the park, to hang out with friends or even at work, you should prepare your own vegan-friendly snacks and beverages and have them with you. This way not only will your budget be safe, but you will also ensure you are eating healthy.

7. In the end, you can always grow your own food. If you are the type of person that cares where your food is coming from, growing your own food is not a bad idea. You will be the one who is in total control of the development of the plant. You will always know what you are consuming. You can also accidentally discover that you love gardening and it may become a new hobby.

8. Take care of what supplements you are buying. The supplement industry can be a tricky one. They strive for-profit and will often sell you things you really don't need. Their advertising is highly effective, but the product is nothing more than sugar water with a placebo effect. However, protein powder is a different story. They are nutrition punches and are a must-have for vegan bodybuilders. In previous sections where we

discussed calories, macronutrients, and their importance we learned that protein would help you recover, repair and build your muscles. Protein powders are also extremely convenient for easy preparation, even when you are on the go. Be careful to always buy vegan-friendly protein powder and any other supplements you decide to buy.

In order to easily plan your meals, you can always use websites such as eatthismuch.com

This website will provide you with tools and support you need to start your new vegan bodybuilding journey. They focus on healthy eating, planning your meals, shopping, and cooking. *Eatthismuch* is a great help for beginners. For all those who plan to change their diet and who need that little bit of extra push to make the change.

Signing up for this website is free, but you will be given a choice to subscribe and support this little company in the awesome work they do. Subscribing will give you plenty of new features like planning for leftovers, weekly meal planning, family meal planning and many more. The cost is 9 dollars per month, or if you chose to buy a yearly subscription, the price would drop to 5 dollars per month (the prices are given as they were at the time of the writing of this book). This website will help you plan, prepare and progress in your diet. You will be asked to input your dietary goals, preferences, and allergens. You can browse their database of restaurants or prepackaged food retailers. You will also be able to input your favorite recipes or search for some new ideas from their database. You can update your detailed nutrition information in real-time. *Eatthismuch* will help you prepare by sending you weekly emails with a complete grocery list, cooking tools needed and cooking instructions. You can always opt to substitute some of the proposed ingredients. You can even set options such as "meals for the whole family" or "meal size". Set your sodium, cholesterol and fiber targets to receive proposals for well-balanced meals and keep track of your diet to get the best possible results.

Summary

There are many challenges a new vegan bodybuilder needs to overcome. The best way to do it is to become aware of them and to approach them equipped with knowledge. In this section, you learned what calories, macro, and micronutrients are and how to properly consume them in order to achieve your desired goals. We showed how simple it is to calculate your TDEE and how to add or restrict calories in order to bulk or cut. You don't have to do the calculations on your own. There are plenty of apps and websites that can help you with this. And in the end, we did pay special attention to discussing the realities of being a vegan on a budget, as veganism is still considered one of the more expensive lifestyles. Plan your meals properly and ahead of time to get the best results. There is even a website that can help you with this planning so you will have more time and energy to focus on your workout.

CHAPTER 4

You're At the Gym...
Now What Do You Do?

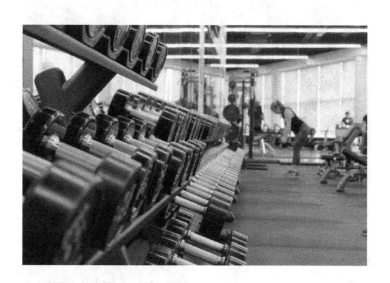

Now that you've mastered the basics and know more about nutrition, we can get to the core of bodybuilding: the gym. In this chapter we are going to discuss choosing the right gym for you, and how to work out. You will learn what types of exercises there are and which ones you should go for in the beginning, but you will also learn how to improvise if you are traveling and you don't have access to any gym.

How to Choose the Best Gym

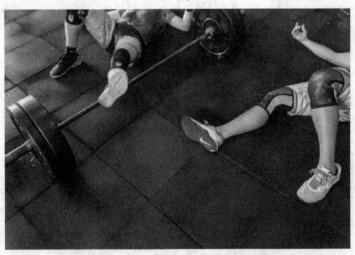

Choosing the gym is the first big step you will take when you start out bodybuilding. Naturally, you always have the option of working out at home or setting up your personal gym if you have enough space and if finances allow it. However, the best option is without a doubt going to the gym because that particular environment will, in fact, motivate you much more.

With that being said, there are many gyms to choose from. Some advertise themselves as gyms for women, or powerlifters, bodybuilders, and so on. Let's discuss what you should look for when choosing the optimal gym.

Budget

The first concern for most people is, of course, the cost of going to the gym. Many bodybuilders and people who look to get fit can't afford deluxe memberships, personal trainers and various group exercising events. If you are in this category like most people, don't worry. It doesn't mean that you can't afford a gym membership.

First of all, you should make a list of the gyms in your area and take a look at their offers. Compare the basic memberships as well as other types of memberships. If you're smart and good with research you can find some really good deals.

The first aspect that affects membership price is the season. There are times of the year when all gyms become accessible due to significant discounts. It's during this time when you can talk advantage of serious offers and purchase a half year or even a year membership for half the price it would normally cost you, or even for less. These seasons are during peak gym joining periods of the year, and there are normally two such periods.

The first is whenever students are returning to school. Many of them flock to the nearby gyms and gyms know it, so they prepare good offers to welcome as many customers as possible. The second period is around the New Year. This is the time when nearly everyone makes their New Year resolutions and many of them promise themselves to go to the gym and change their lives for the better. Again, the gyms are aware of this crowd and they take advantage of them, especially knowing that many of them will give up after the first month, even though they paid for several.

If you can hold out with your membership to join around these times, do so, and then purchase a long-term membership at a large discount. However, if you can't wait, you might want to look into the best offer you can get until these seasons start, and then change your membership. Just try to not give in to the temptation of opting for a membership that is longer than a year because you might end up disliking the gym for various reasons, or you might move, or find something better. Generally speaking, you shouldn't opt for anything longer than a year. In addition, you should always avoid most extra benefits that the gym is trying to push unless you are specifically looking for them. Remember that you're dealing with a business, and a salesman's job is to sell, no matter whether you need it or not. So, don't give in to pressure, stick to your budget and fulfill your needs.

Members

Another important factor that will affect your decision is the type of members that the gym caters to. There are gyms that target women specifically, or competitive bodybuilders, kickboxers, and so on. These gyms usually build programs around the main group. For instance gyms for seniors might hold a lot of aquatic classes because such exercises aren't rough on the joints. Some gyms may also focus mostly on classes like Zumba and Kangoo jumps and have a very limited bodybuilding section or even none at all.

In addition, if you are a woman, you might also want to check out gyms for women only. Large men dropping weights and grunting every few seconds may not create a comfortable atmosphere. Some women feel intimidated by that kind of behavior. Others feel like some men like to stare at them while working out, therefore objectifying them or putting pressure on them and the way they look.

Lastly, you should research the approximate number of members a gym has. These days you can find out how crowded a particular gym is just by using Google. Knowing the peak times of the gym and how many people frequent it is important because you don't want to waste more than 10 minutes waiting in line to finally have access to a bench or a particular machine. This also leads us to the next important point, gym equipment.

Equipment

When you gather a list of viable gyms you also need to consider the type of equipment they have and see whether they have plenty of it. After all, you don't want to stand in line with four other people trying to do a set of bench presses. Furthermore, depending on the type of gym, it might be missing some machines or type of equipment.

The first type of gear you should look for is the free weights category. This includes dumbbells, which are the most basic type of equipment that you will be using often. So make sure they have plenty of dumbbells of all weights.

In addition, you should look at how diverse their weight machines are. There should be multiple machines that are used for each muscle group. Some of them can usually be modified in a few seconds to serve several muscle groups. This will allow you to adapt the machine to different exercises and waste less time changing equipment. Just make sure you can find a few images of the equipment or go to the gym and give it a quick inspection. You don't want to go to a gym that is barely maintained, and the equipment looks like it's going to disintegrate if you touch it.

Finally, as a bodybuilder, you will also need cardio machines. You don't need to be a big fan of cardio exercises, however, they are necessary to some degree, depending on your goals. At the very least you can use them to quickly warm up and get the blood pumping before you start lifting. Some gyms have a limited number of cardio machines however, and some of them are also badly maintained. Make sure that the treadmills are modern, that you can also incline them, and that the bikes are in good condition. Other machines like rowing machines are a bonus, but they aren't necessary unless you really like that type of exercise.

Accessibility, Cleanliness and More

Having easy and convenient access to a gym is ideal. While taking everything else we discussed into account, you should first check all the options you have within walking distance of your home. If that's not an option, make sure the gym is reasonably close. The further away it is, the less likely you will go to the gym, especially early in the morning or after a day of hard work. Another option would be a gym that is close to where your job is. That way, you can always exercise right after your working hours before going home, or when you're on your way to work if that's what you prefer.

No matter the location of the gym, the hours of operation are also very important. If you want to go to the gym before going to work, you need to make sure your gym is open at those hours. Or what if you work night shifts, or you're simply a night owl and you rest most of the day. You need a gym that is open 24/7 so that you can plan your workout as flexible as possible. Going to the gym should be fun, or at least tolerable, not frustrating and a chore.

Finally, cleanliness should also be at the top of your decision-making factors. Gyms are places where bacteria can easily spread because various people come and go all the time, use the equipment and leave their sweat behind. This might sound really gross, but don't allow it to put you off from going to the gym. All you need to do is make sure that the gym has staff that is dedicated to cleaning the rooms and the equipment regularly. In addition, there should be towels and sanitizing solutions available for people to wipe the equipment after using it. Keep in mind that sometimes towels aren't provided, but gyms should at least have a "bring your own towel" policy.

Gym Etiquette

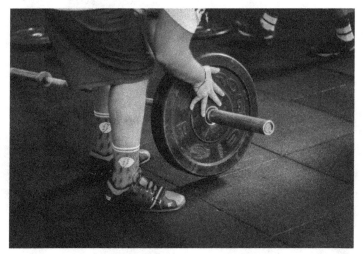

So, you've chosen the right gym for you and now you're ready to get started. However, there's one last detail, and that is gym etiquette. All gyms have an unwritten code of conduct and if you don't know how to follow it, you will become "that guy", and you don't want that. With that being said, here are some of the major rules you should follow no matter to what gym you subscribe:

1. Ask politely: One of the rudest and most annoying things anyone can do at the gym is heading to the rack where someone is doing squats or bench presses, and just grabbing a weight plate. Not to mention it's dangerous because you might distract that person or knock into him or her while they're lifting heavy weights. So make sure to always ask if you can use the same machine or if you can take some weights.

2. Return the dumbbells: If you haven't gone to the gym yet, the first time you do you will without a doubt notice a guy with around six different dumbbells surrounding him, or one huge 50kg dumbbell just lying in the middle of the gym. Please don't be the one who does that. Grab a pair of dumbbells, use them, return them. Simple. Always return any piece of equipment in general and don't just hoard everything for yourself. It makes everyone around you hate you on the spot, even if they may not show it.

3. Unload: Eventually, you will progress significantly, and you will be able to lift a lot of weight. When that time comes, you are going to put a lot of weight plates on various machines,

especially when working out your legs. Once you're done using that machine, unload all of those weights, or at least most of them and put them back on the rack where they belong. Not everyone can lift 20kg - 30kg plates so please be considerate of others. This is also valid for any equipment in general. Try not to move any equipment away from its designated area, or if you do, make sure to move it back once you're done using it.

4. Clean up: Always bring a towel with you because gyms are packed with bacteria. After all, hundreds of people come in contact with the gear every single day and they sweat a lot. If you're a heavy sweater and that towel isn't enough, use the provided paper towels to wipe the machine after using it. Nobody wants to sit on a bench that still has someone's fresh droplets of sweat.

5. Be respectful and mindful of others: A gym is a busy place and people are lifting heavy weights. Always be aware of your surroundings because bumping into someone or even just brushing over them can cause a serious accident. This also means that if you're waiting for a bench or a

machine to free up, you should stand back at a safe distance.

As you can see most of these rules are easy to follow and they will make a huge difference in your gym experience and how others perceive you. You don't want to be the gym rat that everyone looks at angrily for never returning dumbbells or leaving his sweat everywhere. In essence, respect others and you will be respected as well.

Compound vs Isolation Exercises

Now that you're at the gym and everyone is happy to be around you because you know the unwritten code, let's talk exercises!

Generally, there are two types of exercises, namely compound or isolation exercises. To keep it simple, compound exercises are all about working out multiple muscle groups at the same time. For instance, when performing a squat, you will use most of your body, with the hamstrings, glutes and quadriceps sharing most of the load. This is one common exercise that will place enough pressure on three muscle groups in order to increase their mass. Here are some other examples of compound exercises:

1. Bench presses: Whether you are doing them with a barbell or dumbbells in an inclined, declined, or flat position, this exercise will train your chest muscles, as well as your shoulders and triceps.

2. The deadlift: This is another popular compound exercise because it requires most of your body to perform properly. Deadlifts will train mainly your back muscles, but they will also give your hamstrings and glutes a solid workout. In other words, you can use this exercise to train all of your body's backside muscle groups.

3. The squat: This beloved exercise will train most of your entire body, especially considering that there are several variations. You can perform front squats, split squats, back squats, and a few other types of squats. While most of your muscles will be activated during this exercise, the main muscle group that you will train is the quadriceps. However, calves, glutes, and hamstrings will be under significant pressure as well.

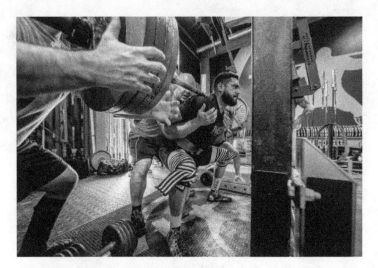

You have probably already noticed that compound exercises have one thing in common, going against gravity. Most exercises that require you to push, pull or squat will have an effect on more than just one muscle group. This makes compound exercises a good way of building strength and stamina, as well as muscle mass, throughout your body.

On the other hand, we have isolation exercises that focus mainly on one single muscle group. Keep in mind that other muscles will also be used, however, only to a small degree. With that being said, here are some of the most common isolation exercises:

1. The dumbbell fly: This exercise will train the chest muscles. However, due to the nature of the

exercise, the shoulders are also under pressure to some degree. This doesn't mean that you are training them, but you run the risk of injuring them if you are using too much weight.

2. Lateral raise: This is probably the best training exercise for your lateral deltoids and you will always see someone performing them.

3. Biceps curls: This is a straightforward exercise that everyone uses to build up their biceps. You can't have a biceps training routine without doing some curls.

4. Calf raises: This is one of the most efficient ways of isolating the calves and working them out. Keep in mind that if you won the genetic lottery you could have nicely developed calves without working out a day in your life. However, if you're not one of the lucky few, you will have to train them or you will end up having a bulky upper body and toothpicks for legs. You don't want that.

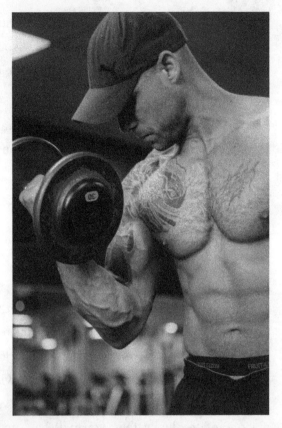

As you can see, isolation exercises are completely different from compound exercises, especially when it comes to form and motion. Basically, everything that involves curling, raising or extending your arms or legs will isolate one of your muscle groups. These exercises are best performed with slightly lighter weights than what your maximum lifting capability is, and by performing a higher number of reps per set.

The bottom line is that both types of exercises come with their benefits and you shouldn't ignore either of them. Even if you feel like you should target your muscles specifically by relying on isolation exercises, you should still incorporate some compound exercises for overall strength and mass. There's more to the human body than specific muscle groups.

Progressive Tension Overload

Deciding what to do at the gym and how to exercise can be quite confusing. Every person has his or her own goals and they depend on a variety of factors. Your diet and exercise list can easily differ from everyone else. This can make you frustrated and lead you to begin the habit of constantly switching to different routines and regimens thinking that it's your fault you don't see any gains. However, if you do this, you are going to waste a lot of time because nothing is consistent. Remember, the key to bodybuilding is having patience and being consistent. This brings us to another piece of the greater puzzle, namely progressive overload.

The idea behind evolving in this sport and making progress is that you need to increase the amount of stress you're subjecting your muscles to. Over time, your muscles grow, become bigger and stronger, therefore the weight you're lifting will no longer have much effect on them. In order to grow strength and muscle mass, you need to challenge your body constantly. Training must be progressive. If you don't progress, you will reach a bottleneck from which you will never escape because your body is already fully adapted. It doesn't matter whether you're increasing the amount of protein and other nutrients if all you do is lift the same weight every single month. This is why you need to implement the idea of progressive overload into your exercising routine.

So how can you progressively overload your muscles? Let's say it's chest day and you're usually doing three sets of ten reps of bench presses with a weight of 100 pounds. Increase that weight to 110 pounds and try your best. You will probably manage to do a set, or two, or maybe just half a set. That's ok. You can start the exercise with a higher weight and then gradually lower it back to 100 pounds. This is already progress. Next week, you will try again and most likely you will do better, even if it's just a few extra reps or even a whole set. Then the next week repeat the same process. After a few weeks, you will find yourself doing three sets of ten reps with 110 pounds on a regular basis. When that happens, it's time to throw in another 5 or even 10 pounds and restart the process.

This method should be applied to all exercises. However, you should never sacrifice your technique or form to lift those extra pounds. Many beginners get too eager to see that progress, so they throw more weight on the bar, weight that they can't correctly lift. For instance, it's common to do this with bench presses, and this leads the bodybuilder to using his back muscles to compensate for the lack of power in his or her pectorals and shoulders. Never do that! If you can't do the exercise correctly using the right muscle groups, then you are using too much weight. Not being honest with yourself can lead to serious injuries, so always be conscious about what you can do and what you can't. There's no shame in it, even if you see those around you lifting 100 pounds more than you. You will get there eventually through gradual progression not by looking for shortcuts.

Sample Training Program

Let's start training!

First, make sure to start with a warm-up session. It doesn't have to take long, but the general idea is that you need to warm up in order to avoid all sorts of injuries. This is especially true when it comes to compound exercises.

As mentioned earlier, compound exercises will put pressure on several muscle groups. This means that you will activate several muscles at once and you are also going to stress a number of joints. Because of this, you should dedicate at least 10-15 minutes to warm up. If you're mostly doing isolation exercises, then you can cut the warm-up session down to 5-10 minutes. With that being said, here's how you should warm-up before training:

1. Start with cardio. Generally, five minutes is enough to get the heart racing and the blood pumping. You don't need more than that to loosen up. However, some bodybuilders like to perform their entire cardio routine before weight lifting. Yes, cardio is important for bodybuilders as well, so we'll talk about that soon.

2. Stretch your muscles and do some bodyweight exercises. A good warm-up before lifting weights is working with nothing more than your own weight. In addition, you could use a stretch band and pull it apart to get your shoulders ready.

3. Now you're ready to start your first exercise, but don't do it with full weight. For instance, if the goal is to bench 120 pounds for three sets, you

should start by doing several warm-up sets. Start by doing 10 reps with 40 pounds, then do another set with 60 pounds, then a shorter 90-pound set with 6-8 reps. This should be enough.

4. Once you finish your warm-up sets, you can start benching with the heavy weights.

Keep in mind that you don't need to perform the warm-up sets before every weightlifting exercise, just the first one in order to engage your muscles and joints.

Now let's plan your weekly workout. There are many ways to do this and every bodybuilder has his or her own schedule and preferences. As a beginner, you shouldn't complicate yourself too much, so let's take a look at a basic plan that is great for getting started and later you can customize it as you learn and experience more:

1. Monday is upper body day: Start with a round of incline bench presses. Three sets with 8 reps each should do the trick. Because this is quite a demanding exercise, make sure to rest two to three minutes between sets. Continue with three sets of dumbbell rows. Again, the same amount of reps and rest. Make sure in between exercises to hydrate yourself properly. Next up, we have three sets of dips, followed by three sets of lateral

pulldowns using a wide grip. At this point, you can reduce your breaks between sets down to two minutes max. Then continue with three sets of side lateral raises, with around 12 reps per set and further reduce the break to a minute and a half max. At this point you will probably be tired, so reduce the last two exercises to only two sets each. You will perform the tricep extension and the barbell curls to finish off, again with short breaks.

2. Tuesday is lower body day: Start with the squats and perform three sets with eight reps each. Since this is the first exercise and it is quite demanding you should rest for three minutes between sets. Continue with leg curls, leg presses and calf raises for three sets each, and only two-minute breaks. Finally, do some abs with 10 to 15 reps per set.

3. Wednesday is rest day: It's important to take a day off to rest and recover fully. Healing takes time, so don't work out every single day or you will end up injuring yourself.

4. Thursday is upper body day: Start with the overhead barbell press and do three sets of eight reps. Continue with three sets of chin-ups, dumbbell bench presses, cable rows, and chest

flies. Then finish off with two sets of triceps pushdowns and hammer curls.

5. Friday is lower body day: Start your day with three rounds of deadlifts, followed by leg presses, leg curls, calf raises and two rounds of abs.

6. Saturday and Sunday are both rest days.

An alternative to this would be following the same pattern, but taking a break on Tuesday, Thursday, and Sunday.

Is Cardio Really Important?

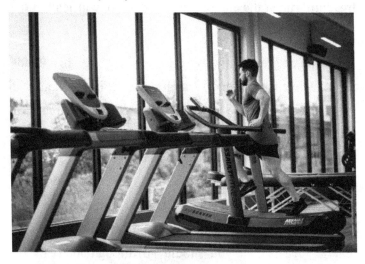

Yes! The heart is a muscle as well and as a dedicated bodybuilder, you need to train as well for long-term health and progress. This means that when you aren't at the gym you should perform some intensive cardiovascular activities. However, if you prefer going to the gym, you can introduce a cardio training schedule into your bodybuilding schedule. All you really need is 30 minutes of activity. You can do yoga, pick up boxing, go jogging, riding a bike, and so on.

Successful cardio doesn't have to be highly intensive. But it is important for overall health, and it can serve as a warm-up session to your weight lifting regimen. In addition, you can also finish your workout with cardio. Some bodybuilders prefer to leave the 20-30 minutes treadmill run at the end of their workout day instead of the beginning.

Another great option is the HIIT cardio. This stands for high-intensity interval training, and it is best suited if your goal is to lose weight. HIIT cardio is great for burning fat at a faster rate without affecting the muscles too much. Remember that when you lose weight you also lose some muscle mass because that's how the body burns fuel during a caloric deficit. However, HIIT cardio will cause you to lose less of that precious muscle mass. The general idea is that you should go through intervals of high-intensity training that pushes your body to the limit for a brief period of time. For instance, on the treadmill, you could comfortably run for 30 seconds and then sprint as fast as you can for another thirty, then repeat for around 15 minutes or more if you can. HIIT cardio is great, but it can be demanding and you might have to gradually work your way up.

Training on the Go

A lot of bodybuilders, especially beginners, have problems when they're away from home and their gym. They find excuses not to work out because they're away and there's nothing they can do. It's easy to end up with this mindset, especially when you find a nice gym and you actually love spending time there. However, this attitude can easily set you back, or even worse make you quit your new habits. So let's avoid all that by learning how to train on the go.

Since you are probably traveling for work or vacation most of the time, you should consider high-intensity workout routines that require only your own body weight and maybe a resistance band that doesn't take much packing space. This kind of workout can keep your body from losing progress, while also not requiring a lot of your precious traveling time. We are talking about a 30-minute workout.

The idea is to perform supersets. You are going to take three different exercises and chain them together. This means you will do a set of one exercise, followed by a set of another, and a set of another, then rest before repeating the superset. Here's an example of such a workout:

1. Minutes 1-10: Three rounds of supersets of squat jumps, bicycle crunches, and push-ups. Take a very short break in between each superset, around 1 minute.

2. Minutes 10-20: Three rounds of supersets of burpees, lunge jumps, and plank. Don't forget to rest between the supersets.

3. Minutes 20-30: Three rounds of supersets of squats, double crunches, and mountain climbers.

If you are really pressed for time, you can reduce this routine to a 20-minute workout by cutting one set from each superset. This way you keep the intensity up and you will really work out those muscles. Such a short workout might not seem like much, but once you go through it you will be exhausted.

Take note, that during similar workouts that don't involve any weights it is very easy to ignore the back muscles. Most of these exercises don't use them, so you will need to buy some kind of rubber bands or resistance bands. In essence, you need something on which you can pull.

Rest Days

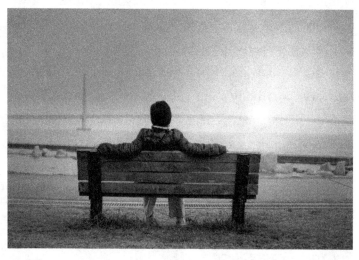

After all the hard work you put in the gym, you would think that the easiest days are the rest days. Wrong. You'll see that once you get in the habit of working out and seeing changes from week to week, rest days become a chore. Many bodybuilders start thinking that rest days are wasted days when they could do more and increase their development at an even faster rate. That mindset could lead to overtraining yourself on a daily basis and then injuring yourself. Rest days are crucial, but in order to force yourself to understand that, you need to know why they are so important to growing muscle mass.

Diet and weight lifting are not enough to grow in a healthy manner. You need time to recover. Muscles need to heal. Therefore, you need to give it time otherwise you will never work out at peak efficiency and you will reach plateaus which will prove to be hard to push through. By recovering properly, your body's strength and endurance will adapt and improve after each session. Without recovery, your body's muscular system, nervous system, and even immune system will put you at risk. The recovery process simply gives the body enough time to adapt to new demands. Only by adapting will you be able to lift more and grow more. This process also involves a healthy dose of sleep.

Get Your Beauty Sleep

Sleep is the best when it comes to rest. A good night of sleep is necessary, especially for bodybuilders. Sleep produces growth hormones, as well as protein synthesis if you consume protein before going to bed. This is important for fixing damaged muscle fibers and conditioning your muscles.

Sleeping at least 8 hours per night is vital, and eating before bed is important. Now, you might think this sounds crazy because you've always heard that you shouldn't go to bed with a full stomach because that will make you gain weight. That is true because during sleep we don't burn many calories. However, if your goal is to build muscle mass, you need to eat protein in particular in order to trigger the protein synthesis in your body.

When you sleep, your body knows that it will go through a period of starvation, so it's going to break down some of the muscle mass into amino acids in order to supply itself with what it needs to repair damaged cells and heal tissue. By eating before bed you will counteract this process because you will be providing everything needed. Some professional bodybuilders even like to wake up in the middle of the night to have a quick meal in order to provide the body with optimal nutrition levels to prevent weight loss.

While you can keep yourself from eating before bed if your goals aren't to build muscle, but lose some fat instead, you still need to sleep properly. The brain and the body need time to recover. Organ cells, muscle fiber, and brain cells are replaced and fixed during this process. Without it, your health can suffer significantly over time. So do not ignore the importance of sleep and quality rest.

Summary

Working out is challenging and without knowing where to start, it can be quite scary for a beginner. So start by choosing the right gym that suits your needs as well as your budget, learn the rules and get to work. Bodybuilding is a lifestyle and the gym is like a club with its own rules. You need to adapt to the gym and perform your exercises correctly in order to go there with a smile on your face. Bodybuilding doesn't have to feel like work, it can be fun, which is why so many become addicted to iron. So make sure to pace yourself, be patient with yourself, and know when to stop for some rest.

CHAPTER 5

Bodybuilding Contest Basics

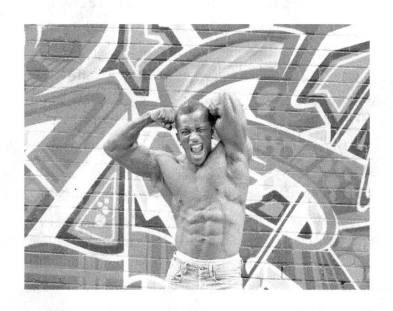

Once you start getting in shape, you should start considering contests. They can be fun, you will meet a lot of people just like you and make friends, and a bit of competition will fuel your drive even more. But how do you plan for bodybuilding contests?

Which Contests Should You Join?

You should already start searching for competitions in your area in advance while you're training. Based on your personal goals, you can choose a contest based on where it is, how large it is and when it is organized. In essence, the best thing about planning for such a contest is that you set yourself a goal that you need to meet. So give yourself plenty of time by already making plans for the off-season.

Getting Ready Pre-Contest

During this phase your goal shifts from building muscle mass to looking good for the upcoming competition. This means that your priority will no longer be strength and muscle mass. That's the off-season, or as some people like to call it, the "bulking" phase. During the pre-contest phase, the purpose is to eliminate as much body fat as possible without losing too much muscle mass. That is why this phase is also commonly known as "cutting". Simply put, the purpose is to look good.

To get ready for contests you will need at least four months. Losing fat rapidly is possible, but it comes with serious consequences like losing too much muscle mass, strength, and significantly slowing down your overall progress.

Since this phase is all about fat loss and maintaining muscle mass, we need to tweak the diet first. You should first start by reducing your caloric intake by about 200 calories below your maintenance requirements in the first couple of weeks. You will progressively reduce the number of calories again later, but we'll discuss that more soon. What's important is to cut those calories from fats and carbohydrates. You should also eliminate your cheat meals, or have them only once every two weeks. In addition, you should increase the amount of protein you consume by 1 gram for every pound of body weight. Naturally, this also means that you need to eliminate certain foods to make room for more protein. The easiest thing to do is to cut out on rich tropical fruits, and potatoes. With that being said, here's how your diet plan should look during the cutting phase:

1. Off-season: This depends on your goals and your weight, but you should consume around 3000

calories, containing plenty of protein, carbs, as well as fat.

2. First 2 weeks of cutting: Consume the same amount of calories but eat as clean as possible. No more processed foods and no more cheat meals.

3. Weeks 2-4: Cut 200 calories out of your diet by reducing carbs and fat.

4. Weeks 4-7: Cut another 200 calories. By the end of this phase, you will plateau and need another calorie reduction.

5. Weeks 7-10: Cut another 200 calories to reach 2400/day. At this point, you should consume more protein than before, even though you reduced the number of overall calories.

6. Weeks 10-13: Weight loss becomes a problem because the body adapted, so you need to start a process called "carb cycling". Once a week you will eat 3000 calories by increasing the number of carbs you eat. The other 6 days in the week you will be eating as low as 2000 calories with a low amount of carbs.

7. Weeks 13-16: Continue cycling but with lower amounts of calories. On a high day reduce to 2800 and on the low days reduce to 1800.

While the diet is what affects your bodyweight the most during the cutting phase, you also need to make a change to your workout routine. If you're doing HIIT cardio at least twice a week, you will need to increase it to four times a week. In addition, you should add another 30 minutes of regular, steady cardio to each workout, preferably at the end of the training session. This way you should eliminate body fat in no time.

In addition to the diet and training, you will also have to focus on tanning and practicing various bodybuilding poses. Tanning should be pretty easy since most gyms provide such services, however, for poses you should hire a personal coach or a trainer at the gym where you're working out.

The Show is Finished... Now What?

Going on the stage as a bodybuilder takes a lot of work and dedication, but coming off of it also takes some work.

Some bodybuilders like to go all-in after the competition and eat all of their favorite meals, including fast food. Some binge like this for days, while others even for weeks. This can be a slippery slope if you aren't careful.

When you're done with the cutting phase, your metabolism is slow because it has adapted to a near-starvation diet. This means if you start going back to your off-season diet from the start, you will rapidly gain weight. The solution to this problem is to diet in reverse.

You need to gradually increase the number of calories you consume, just like you reduced them. All you need to do is take the cutting diet and do it in reverse. Every couple of weeks, increase the intake of calories. This includes slowly eating more carbs and fat. After around 3 months, you should be back to normal, consuming 3000 calories a day without gaining fat.

Now that you're back to normal, you need to plan your next goal. Celebrate your progress, seek new ways of improving and set the goals you want to achieve next year.

Summary

Joining a professional bodybuilding competition can be quite intimidating. You might think that you aren't good enough or that you don't belong there, but you're wrong. Anyone can participate and other bodybuilders will congratulate you on taking that step because they all know what it takes to enter a competition. So prepare yourself in advance and look at your chosen bodybuilding competition as the goal for the year. Get ready by following the right cutting diet, practice the bodybuilding poses, and celebrate your personal success even if you don't win!

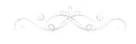

CHAPTER 6

Lifestyle and FAQs About Vegan Bodybuilding

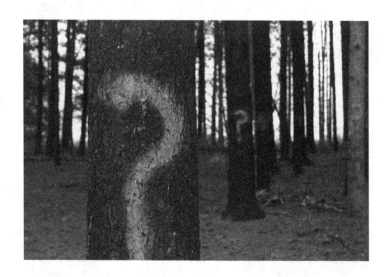

If you are new to veganism, bodybuilding, or both, there must be a thousand questions swirling in your mind. Sometimes, we are overwhelmed with information and it is not easy to find the right one at the moment when we need it. This chapter can serve you as a constant reminder through your journey in building your better self. With trying to answer some of the most frequently asked questions, we hope you will not just get the weapons to combat your own doubts and insecurities, but also you will learn how to defend from others, who might see your new way of life as a threat to them.

Why do vegans in the fitness industry get so much hate?

There is a simple answer to the first and most asked question. It's fear. The western culture is indoctrinated in the opinion that if we are not eating meat, we will not get all of the much-needed nutrients for our day to day lives. It is even worse when it comes to sport, as for many years, a meat-based diet was seen as the only sustainable diet for a competitive fitness career. The fear that you will do yourself more harm than good by just eating a plant-based diet is engraved in the minds of western society. However, there is also the fear of the unknown. People are simply not acquainted with new studies and new examples of benefits of vegan diet. They are not yet aware of what veganism actually is, let alone of its role in fitness. The other possible answer would be guilt. Vegans may make people feel guilty. Even the simple fact that you chose to be a vegan may be received by others as a condemnation of their own choices. In the fitness industry, this is even more pronounced as bodybuilders and athletes are used to thinking that it is a meat-based diet that pushes their performance to the top. Challenging their way of life, and their choices will always lead to at least some degree of resentment. However, things are changing, and the word of veganism in fitness is getting out there. Today we have not just various studies confirming that the fitness life on plant-based diet is possible, and even recommended, but we also have examples in various athletes who either started as vegans or changed their diet preference somewhere during their career.

Is working out twice a day good or bad?

Working out twice, or even more times a day was usually thought to be reserved for professional athletes who are preparing for a competition or a specific event. In today's busy life, with work, school, family and other obligations, it is hard to find enough time to work out once a day, let alone twice. However, the concept shouldn't be dismissed so easily. If you have time and energy, there might be benefits in it. Before diving into a discussion of the pros and cons of working out twice a day, it is important to say that it is safe. As long as you are well aware of what you are doing and you are following a well-structured work-out plan, you are in no danger of injuring yourself. Getting enough rest in between work-out sessions is also very important to avoid injuries. Let's not forget about sleep as possibly the most important factor of rest. A good diet and staying hydrated will also help you recover faster and prepare your body for a second work-out session of the day. As for the benefits of working out twice a day, there are plenty. You will help your muscles build up strength and mass faster as you are sending the signal to your body to develop twice as often. If you are in the process of weight-loss, working out twice a day will burn even more calories than just one session. The blood pressure will be reduced with more exercises you do, and the levels of bad cholesterol will go down. Another great benefit is that insulin sensitivity will go up as well as the levels of good cholesterol. When it comes to bodybuilding, lifting twice a day is extremely beneficial as protein synthesis and anabolic output is greatly increased helping you gain more strength and muscle mass. In general, if you workout in the morning, it's a great way to energize yourself for the start of the day. Reap the workout in the evening and you will lift the stress from your mind and body and prepare it for a good night's rest.

Of course, there can be some drawbacks from working out two times a day and it is really important to take precautions and do it safely. You are putting yourself at risk of straining neuromuscular systems and increasing the possibility of injuries. It is possible for your two workout sessions per day will be followed by pains and aches that will disturb your sleep. This is why it is very important to let your body fully rest before engaging in the second session of the day. It is also noted that some people are prone to mood changes due to overtraining and that their immune system suffers, making them prone to developing seasonal illnesses like colds and flu. Working out may be beneficial but be cautious about it and take steps to prevent any drawbacks that could follow.

How do I get enough Vitamin E on a vegan diet?

Vitamin E is an essential vitamin, which means, it cannot be produced in our bodies, and we have to absorb it through food or supplements. It is also considered a "wonder vitamin" as its health benefits are numerous. It is a complex of chemicals that includes tocotrienols and tocopherols commonly united under the name Vitamin E. It is famous for its antioxidant powers capable of neutralizing free radicals making us healthier in our day-to-day lives. In bodybuilding and in fitness in general, Vitamin E has a second role to play. It has an amazing ability to reduce inflammatory disorders such as muscle soreness and cramps. However, the overall benefits that Vitamin E brings to a well-balanced organism are not to be ignored. One of the main reasons why cardiologists recommend its intake is its ability to prevent the development of atherosclerosis (plaques of bad cholesterol accumulated in the walls of arteries). New studies are showing that the intake of Vitamin E needs to double from what was the recommended daily dose. New recommendations for both men and women are 15 mg of Vitamin E per day. However, this dosage is based only on dietary sources. To prevent the damage caused by free radicals, even more Vitamin E is needed in our system. The recommendation is approximately 400 IUs, a number that cannot be achieved by simple diet intake of the vitamin. Supplements are needed if you want to benefit from the fullest potential of this "wonder vitamin". However, do not forget that it is important to take in this vitamin through food, do not rely only on supplements.

Some vegans find it challenging to reach daily doses of required Vitamin E, but foods such as seeds, nuts, wheat germ and oils such as sunflower, safflower, rapeseed, corn, and soy. Note that olive oil does not have enough Vitamin E to be considered a good source of it. Vitamin E can also be found in vegetables with meaty green leaves such as spinach, turnip greens, asparagus, and broccoli. Even some plant-based kinds of milk are enriched with Vitamin E and its intake should not be a problem for bodybuilders who are on a vegan diet.

What are Oxalates?

Simply put, oxalates are molecules that prevent the absorption of calcium. They also play a role in the creation of kidney stones. Vegans are familiar with oxalates because our food is rich with them. They cannot be found in the food of animal origin, only in plants. However, the studies done on people who are planning their diet around vegetables showed that vegans actually have a lower occurrence of kidney stones. There are other factors that influence the formation of calcium deposits in kidneys other than oxalates and vegans are in no more risk than any other human being. The trouble is that there is a belief that many other illnesses are caused by absorbing too many oxalates. Diseases such as interstitial cystitis, vulvodynia, depression, fibromyalgia, depression, autism and many more are linked with the presence of oxalates in the organism, but there are no extensive studies done to support such beliefs. People do report feeling better overall if they reduce their intake of oxalates and it wouldn't be such a bad idea to be aware of foods with a high content of this molecule. Not all plant-based foods contain oxalates, and some have them in much lesser amounts than others. Plants that are known to contain high amounts of oxalates are spinach, beets, beet greens, sweet potatoes, peanuts, and rhubarb. There are precautionary steps vegans can take to minimize their intake of oxalates. Boiling their greens and discarding the water is an excellent idea. Eat high calcium foods or take calcium supplements with your meals. If you have a history of calcium-oxalate stones in kidneys, you should take calcium citrate as prevention and minimize intake of added fructose and sodium.

What is the best time to work out?

Some people swear that working out at exactly 6 am is the best service you could do for your body. Others will say the same for an evening work-out session. The truth is, they are both right, or wrong if you prefer. There is no such thing as the perfect time for work-out, as it is an individual thing. It depends on what kind of person you are. Some people simply love working out in the morning as it gives them a nice boost for the rest of the day, others cannot even fathom breaking a sweat before noon. Basically, the time of day you choose for the exercise does influence how you will feel about it, and how you will feel after it. While morning workouts can indeed boost you and give you the power needed to go through the day, some people are just not wired for it, and they prefer to start the day slowly. However, evening exercise, be it a work-out or a simple jog around the block, will relieve you of stress accumulated during the day and prepare your body for sleep and the rest phase. What is important is to choose a time of day that you are able to stick with. In this way you will develop the habit of working out at the same time, and in time it will become a routine. What you could do as an individual is to listen to your body, acknowledge if you are a morning type of person, evening, or even mid-day, and respect the wishes of your body. Experiment, if needed, and try working out at different times of a day. This will help you determine which type of person you are and what time of day suits you best for exercises. If you discover you are not, for example, a morning person but you don't have the time for work-out during the day due to obligations, do not worry. It is easy to program your body to start the day by working out. Simply be persistent and work out always at the same time of day to create a habit.

How to eat right while traveling?

Many vegans find it challenging to travel and keep eating healthy as the comfort of their own kitchen is lost. But there are ways to keep your healthy vegan diet going even if you are on a business trip or a vacation with friends or family. Busy schedules sometimes won't allow you to prepare your own meals or eat what you crave the most, but little sacrifices do go a long way. Here are some tips on how to stay on a healthy vegan diet while traveling:

1. Bring plant food on your trip and pack it in ample amounts. The easiest and most convenient foods to pack for a trip are nuts, fruits, seeds and bars. However, don't shy away from packing prepared foods such as hummus, avocado rolls, or veggie sandwiches. If packed properly and kept at the right temperature, they are an excellent source of nutrients during your journey. Prepare convenient packages for food and follow the rules and regulations depending on the type of transport you are taking. For example if you are flying, some

companies have strict rules about how food must be packed for a plane ride.

2. Research your food options at your destination on time. Whether you are staying at a hotel, Airbnb or a friend's house, it is important to know in time whether you will have access to a fridge, a vegan-friendly restaurant, a farmer's market and so on. Do your research before the trip so you are prepared and well aware of your options.

3. Don't be shy about preparing your own food while traveling. If vegan restaurants are not an option at your destination, you can always plan your stay that will include your own cooking. There are plenty of supermarkets all around the world where you can buy your own ingredients and prepare the food by yourself. Some of them even sell cooked food and many have vegan-friendly meals on the menu.

4. If you are traveling with non-vegans and choosing a vegan restaurant is a no, propose Indian, Thai, Mexican, Japanese or Vietnamese restaurants as alternatives. These are all restaurants with menus that will satisfy both vegans and non-vegans. The cuisine from these countries is mostly plant-based

and offers a large variety of meals that will suit the needs of all your friends.

5. Don't forget that restaurant food always contains larger amounts of salt, sugar, and calories than you would normally eat with your home-cooked meals. Be prepared to put some extra effort into exercising after eating at a restaurant. If nothing else, take the stairs instead of elevators whenever possible. Use your hotel's gym if it's an option or simply exercise in your hotel room.

6. Avoid the temptation of junk food. Many tourist places are packed with stands that will offer a quick snack for tired and hungry tourists. Some even offer vegetarian or vegan options but that doesn't make them any less junk food. They will probably be high in oil and salt amounts, as well as sugars. Lots of travelers love to snack during their trip and vegans are often tempted by bags of potato chips. Instead, think about the alternatives. Buy some fresh fruits or veggies, bananas are great for tiresome walks around tourist places. High in potassium, they will help you fight muscle cramps.

7. If you are limited to buying food at airports, gas stations, trains or ferries, the food can get pretty expensive. Plan ahead and prepare your own packs of food and beverages from home. Sliced apples, bananas, and oranges make a nice, hearty fruit salad, or veggie salad for the road. Bring less expensive homemade snack bars and bring your own beverages. Remember that liquids are not allowed through the airport checkpoints, but once you are through, you can always fill a bottle of your own with fountain water.

These are just some examples of how to prepare a nice, healthy food plan for travel. With time and experience, there is no doubt you will come with your own solutions for some of the problems and challenges you will meet down the road. Please feel free to share them with other vegan travelers, if nothing else, post on social media recommendations for vegan-friendly restaurants that you've discovered and found interesting.

Raw Vegan Bodybuilding, is it worth it?

Raw Vegans are known to research what they consume to the most extreme details. They are well aware of all the nutrients they are putting in themselves and they know exactly what is going on in their body at any given time. There is a persistent myth that you will never be able to intake enough protein in your body as a raw vegan, but it is an easily disproved myth as nuts, seeds and legumes are absolute stars when it comes to protein. Many vegans will say that going raw is the healthiest thing you can do to your body. Combine that with bodybuilding, and you will have the ultimate recipe for health. However, raw food does bring some dangers with it and it's upon an individual to decide whether the benefits of eating raw are worth it. Uncooked food is simply not safe enough unless you have time and energy to devote yourself to getting really good at blending, drying, germinating and dehydrating your own food. Many illnesses are linked to the consumption of raw food and you will have to be extra careful with high-risk fruits and vegetables such as sprouts, raspberries, unpasteurized juices, lettuce, cucumbers and many more. If you are suffering a chronic illness raw veganism is not recommended due to your weakened immune system. The same rule applies to pregnant women, seniors and children. The best thing you could do is educate yourself, learn as much as possible about raw veganism before you indulge in it, and weigh the pros and cons for yourself to see if this lifestyle suits you. To be healthy you must be fit, and bodybuilding will get you there. But you can be fit without being healthy. It

Is intermittent fasting good or bad?

There are numerous studies on rats that showed how intermittent fasting does improve their metabolism, it reduces cholesterol and blood pressure, it helps with weight loss programs and the general health is improved. But those studies are all done on rats. In humans, there are simply not enough studies relevant enough to show how beneficial intermittent fasting is for our own health. What is proven is that it will help with losing extra weight. Combined with the right diet and exercises, it can be the best thing you could do to your body. However, it comes with its own restrictions that can be mind-boggling and extremely tiresome. It is not a simple way of life as you are restricted to eating food in a timeframe of 8-10 hours, followed by 16 hours of fasting. Some people are simply not good enough with rules and limitations and will give in to unhealthy foods after such long periods of fasting, gorging themselves on junk food and low-nutrient meals. If you are a person who easily deals with discipline and rules, somewhat bordering an OCD personality, intermittent fasting can be the right choice with you, and it even works very well with veganism. However, there are some people who are not cut out for it. For example, it can be an extremely dangerous dietary plan for people who suffer from diabetes and are taking insulin. Fasting can also act as a trigger for people who have a history of eating disorders such as anorexia, bulimia or obesity. Pregnant women and those who breastfeed are not allowed intermittent fasting. And lastly, there are people who simply cannot bear to be hungry and in their case intermittent fasting can be torture. People like that will often try, but quickly give up and indulge in old bad habits. For them, some other dietary plans might work better. Intermittent fasting is not a magic pill that solves all the problems, it's just another option in the sea of dietary plans that will help you lose weight and gain muscle mass. For other benefits than simple weight loss, intermittent fasting has no studies done on humans, and only time will tell if there are any major health benefits from it.

What are my blood test results going to be like?

If you are changing your diet, no matter in what way, doing a regular blood test is recommended for the simple reason that it will give you insight on what is going on in your body. Changing the type of foods we are consuming can drastically influence our blood test results. Every person is different, and there are more factors that influence the results of blood work than just a simple diet, but it is a diet that can help us improve our overall health and the results. Because of this, it is important to not try to interpret the test results on your own. Instead, find a doctor you can trust and who is acquainted with your lifestyle, medical and family history. There are some things you should always be on the lookout for as a vegan, such as B12 and D3 vitamins, but other than that, if your diet is well planned and balanced, together with bodybuilding, it should not change drastically, unless you already had some health issues. In that case, you could see bad cholesterol levels going down, while good cholesterol levels are coming up. For vegans, it is extremely important to check on their levels of vitamin B12 as it cannot be found in any plants and it must be taken through supplements. B12 is important as it is required for red blood cell production and for maintaining nerve health. This vitamin also helps with tissue and cellular repair and because of it, it is especially important for bodybuilders. Deficiency of vitamin B12 will lead you to feel overall weakness, tiredness, heart palpitations, numbness of arms and legs, pale skin and mental issues such as depression and lethargy. As for Vitamin D tests, they are important as a prevention of bone diseases, weaknesses, malformation and abnormal calcium metabolism. Generally, Vitamin D we get from the sun, however, vegans who are spending their time mostly indoors or in areas that are deprived of enough sun must take supplements. Vitamin D is fat-soluble and because vegans are generally on a low-fat diet, they are more in danger of suffering the deficiency. Other tests vegans may pay closer attention to are iron, ferritin test, omega-3 index test, folic acid test, lipid profile test, urinary iodine test, etc. If you are on a well-planned, well-balanced vegan diet, these tests will give you guidelines about your health and will remain in optimal ranges. As to how often it is advised for vegans to do blood tests, it depends. If you are just starting a vegan diet, you may want to do one right at the beginning, after six months, and after 12 months. You will observe the changes in your body and watch it grow healthier. It will also give you awesome guidelines on how to improve and adjust your diet. Once you are completely adjusted to the vegan diet and you find your perfect balance, the tests are not even necessary but are advised occasionally, just as for any other person.

Summary

In this chapter the covered topics, in the form of FAQs, are there to remind you of why is it important to be true to what you are trying to achieve, and to also help you with tips and tricks on how to achieve best results. It is important to understand that each organism is a story for itself, and each body may react differently. Get to know your body by experimenting, and don't be afraid to visit a good doctor, as they are there to help you understand what your body is going through, while you are on a journey to improve your lifestyle. Veganism and bodybuilding do go together, no matter what the conventional opinion is. With a carefully planned, balanced program, you will be able to achieve so much more and feel good about yourself, as there will be no moral dilemmas to put obstacles in your way. Veganism is the purest way of life you could grant to yourself and topped with proper exercises and bodybuilding, it is the ultimate recipe for a healthy, long life.

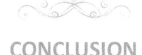

CONCLUSION

There is no secret to bodybuilding and looking fit. It's all about balancing your diet with proper workouts and plenty of rest. That's it! A vegan diet fits perfectly in this equation because it offers all the nutrition the body needs to build strength and muscle mass, while also burning fat.

With the help of this book, you have everything you need to know how to live healthily as a vegan and how to get started in bodybuilding. Focus on nutrition and keep track of everything you eat to make sure you get plenty of protein, vitamins and minerals, and start lifting weights. Anyone can get started in bodybuilding no matter how skinny or fat they are, and no matter your goals, a vegan diet can be customized to no end. There are no excuses, so start your planning today and change your life forever!

Thank you for taking the time to read this guide on vegan bodybuilding. If you found it helpful and enlightening, please take a moment to leave a review.

👀 [Look! Special Offer Currently Available!](#) 👀

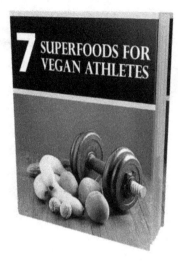

⚠️ <u>Warning</u>: Downloads of this book have been limited to 15 FREE Downloads. Then, the price instantly shoots up to $27 ⚠️

Hurry! Get Your Copy Now by Clicking the Link Below:

➡️ brad-speer.com/special-offer ⬅️

Here's <u>just a fraction</u> of what you'll discover:

- 7 secret superfoods that you had <u>NO IDEA</u> existed!
- A secret superfood to increase the release of testosterone!
- How these foods can enhance your overall health and build muscle too!

...and <u>so much more</u>!!

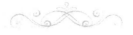

REFERENCES

Chekroud, S.R., Gueorguieva, R., Zheutlin, A.B., Paulus, M., Krumholz, H.M., Krystal, J.H., et al. Association between physical exercise and mental health in 1·2 million individuals in the USA between 2011 and 2015: a cross-sectional study. The Lancet Psychiatry. Vol. 5, iss. 9. p. 739-746. Retrieved from https://doi.org/10.1016/S2215-0366(18)30227-X

Denny, K.G., & Steiner, H. (2009). External and Internal Factors Influencing Happiness in Elite Collegiate Athletes. Child Psychiatry Hum Dev 40, 55. https://doi.org/10.1007/s10578-008-0111-z

Fitschen, P. J., & Wilson, C. (2020). Bodybuilding: the complete contest preparation handbook. Champaign, IL: Human Kinetics.

Hatfield, F. C. (1984). Bodybuilding: a scientific approach. Chicago: Contemporary Books.

Hughes, M. (2000). The composite guide to bodybuilding. Philadelphia, Penn.: Chelsea House Publishers.

Klaper, M. (1998). Vegan nutrition: pure and simple. Paia, Maui, HI: Gentle World, Inc.

LaVelle, G. (2011). Bodybuilding: tracing the evolution of the ultimate physique. Lexington, Kentucky: Romanart Books.

Levine GN, Lange RA, Bairey-Merz CN, Davidson RJ, Jamerson K, Mehta PK, Michos ED, Norris K, Ray IB, Saban KL, Shah T, Stein R, Smith SC Jr; on behalf of the American Heart Association Council on Clinical Cardiology; Council on Cardiovascular and Stroke Nursing; and Council on Hypertension. Meditation and cardiovascular risk reduction: a scientific statement from the American Heart Association. J Am Heart Assoc. 2017;6:e002218. DOI: 10.1161/JAHA.117.002218.

U.S. Department of Health and Human Services and U.S. Department of Agriculture. (December 2015). 2015–2020 Dietary Guidelines for Americans. 8th Edition. Available at http://health.gov/dietaryguidelines/2015/guidelines/

CPSIA information can be obtained
at www.ICGtesting.com
Printed in the USA
LVHW111356030321
680478LV00025B/561